I0477041

Zara's Crippled Son

*A Black Doctor's Struggle
in the Medical Profession*

Nyaba E. Yamusah, M.D.

Copyright © 2015 by Nyaba E. Yamusah, M.D.

Library of Congress Control Number: 2015905174
ISBN: Hardcover   978-1-5035-5917-2
                 Softcover   978-1-5035-5942-4
                 eBook   978-1-5035-5916-5

All rights reserved. No part of this book may be reproduced or transmitted in any form or by any means, electronic or mechanical, including photocopying, recording, or by any information storage and retrieval system, without permission in writing from the copyright owner.

Any people depicted in stock imagery provided by Thinkstock are models, and such images are being used for illustrative purposes only.
Certain stock imagery © Thinkstock.

Print information available on the last page.

Rev. date: 09/01/2015

To order additional copies of this book, contact:
Xlibris
1-888-795-4274
www.Xlibris.com
Orders@Xlibris.com
531833

ACKNOWLEDGEMENT

This book could not have been written without the constant support and encouragement from my wife of twenty-six years, Dilder, and my four children; Mallik, Amina, Adisa and Amal who have had to deal with my tantalizing Bulbia village stories. I wish to thank my only maternal brother, Mr. Zibrim Yamusah, and my sister, Lamisi, who at times had to sacrifice for me to achieve my goal of becoming a doctor. My oldest sister, Azumah, often played the role of my mother when we found ourselves in her house in Wale Wale whenever we were on vacation and did not want to go back to the village. Many thanks also go to my maternal aunt, Lahari, who nursed me back to life after I was bitten by a snake in her house, and my Aunt Asibi who often made sure we had a place to stay overnight any time we were going to Bulbia through Wungu. To all my maternal uncles Goabinaba, Kpanbinaba and Issaku and my paternal uncle Karim— who despite my father's attitude towards him, willingly took us to go back to Wale Wale in the midst of floods without any hesitation— may you all rest in peace. Despite the Wale Wale Local Council's refusal to sponsor me for my secondary school education in Navasco, I enrolled and attained an academic Cocoa Marketing Board scholarship throughout my secondary school education. I wish to thank all the cocoa farmers of Ghana for helping make me what I am today. I would also like to thank all my classmates and teachers, especially Mr.

McDonald in Navasco who helped me tremendously and encouraged me to apply for the National Essay competition.

To the Olson family of Bloomer, Wisconsin, especially my American mother Mrs. Victor Olson, I extend my greatest thanks. The student exchange year was not only enjoyable but challenging and would not have been successful without my American host family. The year would not have been complete without my lifelong friends, Bonnie Doyle and Debbie Feiten. I wish to thank my first year academic advisor at UW-Eau Claire who counseled me on the necessary courses to take as a pre-Med student, even though she didn't think somebody from African could successfully complete a chemistry degree. To all the teachers in UW-Eau Claire who gave grades based on one's color and did all they could to prevent me from attaining a medical education, I thank them because they only increased my desire to become a medical doctor. Dr. Ibrahim Ibrahim of Englewood Hospital was instrumental in my medical externship training and I thank him very much for the teaching and confidence he had in me. I wish to thank Dr. Arnold Rubin as my Fellowship Director in Hematology and Oncology. My final thanks and salutations are reserved for the best mother I could ever ask for. My mother did not follow the norm of throwing her crippled son to the streets of Ghana. She took the blame for everything in order to get me treated and she taught me to never give up in life because failure is a bad option to choose. I lost my mother in 2012 but she is still with me every day. Thanks to my wonderful parents and may God protect them till we get together again. She lived to see her crippled son become a doctor and helping other helpless persons.

I wish to thank Xlibris Publishing for helping get my cry for the improvement of the health care system to all Americans published. I wish to thank Kris Albero, Bernadette Valdez, Lloyd Griffith, Apple Jean, Nancy Summers and numerous others who encouraged me to complete this book.

ABSTRACT.

The main purpose of this book is to describe how a crippled son who could have easily have been left on the streets or killed as the work of the devil, was raised by an uneducated woman; has risen from being raised in a mud hut in Bulbia, a viillage in Ghana to become a sub-specialist in Hematology and Oncology in the United States of America.

It describes the authors journey from childhood, the several medical challenges he goes through and the influence religion plays in his final treatment and ability to walk through Mbazoa. People do not make religion but religion guides us into righteousness. We are fighting wars, bombing each other in this world today in the name of religion. Everyone wants and prays for peace but nobody wants to know why and how each side feels. No body sits at the peace table any more. The United Nations has and continues to fail us as a peace loving and making institution. It is easier to bomb, mame and kill each other all in the name of religion or because of our power. Our inability to discuss, understand and respect each other has resulted in families not being able to talk to their children, children not able to hold friendly discussions or solve disputes between themselves, husbands not able to discuss with their wives and as a result we see dramatic increase in violent crimes and the onslaught of the greater use of the gun as the arbitrator of disputes. The author also demonstrates how the misuse of

our differences be it race, color, religion or nationality has continued
to infiltrate into our healthcare system. The use of black people in
this country in medical experimentation is a known fact. What the
system does not and will not admit today is that this practice still
goes on unabated. Today in most medical teaching institutions in this
country blacks and Hispanics make up the bulk of the people who are
used to teach medical students, Residents and Fellows. They are also
the most disrespected and often the most maltreated human's in our
health care system. The few black and Hispanic doctors can barely be
seen in the Private medical business world where the decision makers
inhabit mainly due to established social, religious and racial divide
that mimics what goes on in society. The black medical professional
cannot get privileges or participate in the teaching of our future
doctors not because they are not qualified or competent but because
of established racism that makes sure that in a Catholic institution
like St. Joseph's Hospital only Italian or Arab physicians make up
the bulk of the teaching core when most of the patients are African
Americans or Hispanic. In disguise of the real reasons, professional
lies and deceit are often used to denigrate people to prevent the
minority professional from attaining privileges in hospitals. Hospital
committees which are to represent the vestiges of democracy are often
limited to certain racial or economic blocks so that they can be used
as weapons against minority groups or against physicians who do not
refer their patients to the committee chairperson or the racial or ethnic
group in question. Hospital committees are often limited to Black
or Brown doctors even if and when one volunteers for them. These
committee positions are offered to black doctors if and only when they
are hired by the institution and conforms to the honor code of their
bosses. Once an employed physician expresses their own opinion as
to how a minority patient is taken care of or other issues within the
institution; lies and false reports are often made to get the physician
out of the institution. The only system that most minority doctors
or other medical professional then relies on is the government jobs
or the army where they are often shipped to participate in wars they
morally do not believe in but have to support their families. What
is the use of going to fight for somebodies freedom and liberation in
another country when as a black man or Hispanic you cannot even get

an application for privileges in a hospital in your own country even when the legal institution requests it to be done.. Excellent physicians have been destroyed not because of malpractice or lack of malpractice insurance and/or incompetence, but through lies, cover-up, making up of documents that don't exist and reporting to State or Regional Medical Boards who often have their friends and/or political and racial allies in the institutions sitting in judgment like a goat being left in front of a lion's den. The American society will eventually immensely be the benefactor if Black and Hispanic medical personnel are incorporated into the hospitals teaching programs and management The practice of medicine is an art and involves the understanding of differences in culture. Imbibing minorities into teaching programs rather than requiring people to take a test to show their competency in minority care will go a long way to reduce the millions and millions of dollars spent on testing instead of speaking or touching the patient and understanding their concerns. Minorities especially blacks are often the sickest, the last to be admitted to hospitals as recently demonstrated in our recent Ebola case involving black patients and they are often the first to be discharged home whether they are better or not to sub-acute care facilities owned by the same institutions that hurried to get them out in the first place. A black doctor who feels that minority patients are often discharged prematurely by the institutions quality management teams or the Insurance company is often categorized and punished for what is morally right. Certain medications are too expensive to be used on minority patients and presccibers cannot use medications such as intravenous gammaglobulin on thrombocytopenic patients because they are too expensive and a prescriber has to show every article available to show that the treatment is indicated. However if the same medication is given to a Caucasian patient no similar cannotions is expressed about the care of the patient. There is consensus in this country that the health of the blacks and Hispanics are the poorest in terms of the high morbidity and mortality Every reason is often given to blame the same people who do not trust the system or are often disrespected. The medical establishment often agrees that something is woefully wrong in a medical system that is gauged the best for a certain part of its populous whilst the minority lives under substandard conditions.

Every reason is often made to explain this in excusable scenario except racism which is still an open sore in our socciety that nobody wants to accept exist in the champion of the free world. . It is unlawful but the conscience of the country has not lived up to the expectations of our laws...

CONTENTS

- Life in America an an AFS International High School Exchange Student and the testing of my Catholic Faith and believes.

- Return to Ghana and G.C.E. 'A' Education in Navasco.

THIRD PHASE OF ZARA'S CRIPPLED SON

- University Education (undergraduate and graduate) in America and my maternal grandmother Amina's funeral.

- The making of Zara's Crippled Son as a Medical doctor and life in the West Indies as a medical student.

- Medical Externship experience in American Hospitals.

- Residency Training in Internal Medicine in Englewood Hospital (NJ) and the onset of H.I.V. and AIDS Epidemic.

- Sub-Specialist training in St. Joseph's Hospital and the establishment of the first Autologous and Allogeneic Bone Marrow Transplantation in New Jersey.

- Working as a Physician Specialist and Consultant in Grenada and my first experience with a Political Medical Directive and Mr. Kwame Toure (Mr. Stokely CarMichael).

- Return to U.S from Grenada and the Completion of my fellowship in Hematology and Oncology.

THE FOURTH PHASE OF ZARA'S CRIPPLED SON.

- Zara's Crippled Son as a Hematologist and Oncologist in Solo Private Medical Practice in Paterson, N.J. and the Struggles of a Blackman in the American Health Care System.

- Obtaining Hospital Medical Privileges in St. Joseph's Hospital, Paterson, N.J.

- Teaching (Non-private) and Non-teaching (private) patients: The role of the Black and Hispanic patient and how Hospital politics influences their care.

- Quality Care Management, Hospital Committees, the Hospital administration and the Black Doctor, Black patients and institutional racism in American Health Care.

- Post Closure of Barnert Hospital, Hospital Monopoly and the Blackballing of Community physicians.

FIRST PHASE OF ZARA'S CRIPPLED SON

Growing up in a Kantonsi household and the Mole-Dagbani Heritage in Ghana, West Africa.

The morning breeze blew across my father's mud hut's window as i strolled from one side of my daddy's hut to the front door of the Naa Zibrim's ancestral compound in Bulbia. This morning breeze during the harmattan season blows cold dusty wind across not only Bulbia but the whole of the West and East Mamprusi Districts of Ghana. The winds originates from the Sahara and are often aided by the White Volta River which is a stone throw from Bulbia in a small fishing village called Bimbini.

Walking around Naa Zibrim's compound and towards the Bulbia marketplace which harbored my youthful playground, it occurred to me that I had made it out of this small village of huts, lizards (which are alleged to represent the re-incarnation animal of the Kantonsi tribe and can be found all over the village) and numerous Dawa Dawa and Shea nut trees into a larger world consisting of skyscrapers, electricity, refrigeration and crime that was not only new but challenging in several aspects..

I had gone back to visit with my family. It seemed to to be a dream but it was real. I was back in my own village, Bulbia, the cradle of the Kantonsi tribe where my family lived till my world changed with challenges and blessings that could not have been imagined.

I was blessed to be born into an educated family. Our household was the only one in a village of about two thousand people who had western style education. Most people in Bulbia are all related. The Kantonsi tribesmen makes up the majority of the villages inhabitants as well as a small number of Mamprusis and Builsa tribesmen. Kantonsi tribesmen can often be identified by three tribal marks on each side of the face or around the navel. The theme song of the Kantonsis is:' Kantonsi belligu piersa ata' signifying the importance of the three tribal marks to the tribe.

I was born in Bulbia in the Northern part of Ghana in the midst of the cold harmattan season when the dust bowls and strong and gentle winds blow from the Sahara plains through the old Ghana-Mali-Songhai Empires where the Mole-Dagbani heritage originated. It is also an area that a lot of slave raids and slave trading was carried out during the period in human history when these inhumane practices were allowed to flourish amongst human brutality that has had a long and lasting impact on black people throughout the whole world which the perpetrators of this evil practise have not yet acknowledged exists.

In this land of history, we had the indigenous owners of the land called the *tingdana* who were later supplanted by the Mamprusi Kingdom, which brought their sophisticated chieftaincy system of rule to dominate the inhabitants of the land and eventually assisted in enslaving some of these smaller tribes through war and other methods of division among tribes.

Whether the Kantonsi tribe was enslaved by the Mamprus's or not was a topic my father and the extended family did not talk about, and as a child in my tribal system, one could not ask questions about matters which were meant for discussion by the elderly. You are too young to understand; was the main excuse the elderly often gave. for not giving answers to questions that were either very dear to them, painful or sexual in nature.

The Mole-Dagbani heritage encompasses most of the current Northern, Upper East, and Upper West Regions of Ghana today where my childhood years was spent.

In the Mole-Dagbani system, there is a centralized system of rule based on Chieftancy (Naam). who have their Advisors and Council of Elders to assist them rule and oversee their territory. The Kantonsi tribesmen are purported to have originated from Toe, now in Burkina Faso and Kpaliwongo in the current Upper West Region of Ghana became the linguist(Masu) (historian/interpreter) and the *lumam* (Islamic religious advisor) to the chiefs who are usually Mamprusis.

The chiefs are generally chosen from what are known as 'gates' (groups of families who are eligible to become Chiefs through heritage). The paramount chiefs such as the *Nayiri* (chief of Nalerigu), *Ya-na* (chief of Yendi) and *Wa- na* (the chief of Wa), choose the sub-chiefs who in turn enskinneds the lesser chiefs such as the Bulibi-Naa(the chief of Bulbia). These institutions are still in place and are more respected in governing the masses of tribesmen with laws and judicial systems that are more respected and honored than our modern political and judicial systems that are often marred in corruption, selfishness, and lack of respect for our indigenous African tradition and culture. Education in this part of Ghana has been hampered by cultural structures that do not want the influence of Western education, but religion in all its forms has also affected Western education and has hampered "development" in these areas.

My paternal grandmother and my Father's Road to Western-Style Education.

My father went to school as a punishment to my paternal grandmother Tiyasi. He obtained the certificate 'A' teaching diploma, which was the highest teaching certificate that could be achieved in the nineteen thirties before college and university education became available in the then Gold Coast, which is now post- independence Ghana. He attended Achimota Teachers Training College in Accra and was one of a few students from the then Northern Territories of the Gold Coast. Like most Africans, my father was brought up in a polygamous family. My paternal grandfather Zibrim, died when my father was about six years of age. In the tradition of the Kantonsi tribe, the widows of the male often remained within the family to ensure that the children were adequately taken care of and remained as part of the community. Generally the widow would remarry one of the older brothers of her deceased husband or a close relative.

It is believed in the Kantonsi tribe that it is the right of every woman to be married and be taken care of by a man. The women had no choice as to the next family they wanted to marry into in most cases.. A single or widowed woman is not an accepted phenomenon in my culture. In my culture, the position of the females on the outside looks like a very chauvinistic one; but when you go into the fabric of the Kantonsi family, the woman is the fulcrum of the family and is well is very well acknowledged and respected for it.

My father was very well educated, thanks to my stubborn and "rule breaking" paternal grandmother. My paternal grandmother, Tiyasi, was a very beautiful woman even when I got to know her at an older age. She was the darling of her village called Prima, which is about thirty miles from Bulbia across the White Volta River.

She apparently was courted by my grandfather, but other contestants who were inhabitants of Prima also participated in trying to secure her heart in marriage.. Nobody could tell me how she made the decision to marry my grandfather Zibrim since it was disrespectful in our culture to ask personal questions. She finally decided to marry my grandfather and then moved from Prima to Bulbia. She bore two boys, and as was the trend in the early part of the twentieth century, education was not only unavailable but many people were reluctant to be imbibed into the Western lifestyle and education.. They did not want to be converted into Christianity since the colonial powers came not only to get slaves and colonize the people but also introduced the Bible and the religious conversions that came with it. The people in my area, which are mainly still animist and Islamic or more a combination of both religious entities, did not want to be converted into the Western culture.

My father's induction into the Western culture and lifestyle began about a year after my paternal grandfather died.

As explained before, it was the policy of the tribal customs for the children of a widow to remain in the paternal household, and it was expected for the woman to remarry in the same family. My grandmother (*nyapoa*) Tiyasi, when I got to know her, was very light skinned, with gray long hair. She was very beautiful.

She was very open minded and enjoyed giving the grandchildren some paddle slaps in the buttocks, which sounded louder than they hurt. I was actually very afraid of my grandmother because she was often called a witch by outsiders. She liked to be by herself and did not cover her long gray hair unlike other women in the village who were culturally and religiously bound to do so.

She was very proud of her two sons since it meant that her sons' generations were going to be extended or perpetuated. People would try several times to get a male in the family if they did not have one already. She deemed herself lucky. She still in her mind often wanted to have a daughter who would stay at home with her and help her out in her compound, but that was not to be. My grandmother was often alone and seemed to enjoy it. However, she stood her grounds in a tribal and Islamic culture where women were not expected to express themselves much more to be stubborn at the same time. Her stubbornness came to a climax one year after my grandfather's death when she refused the Cultural norm of remarrying the family's household. She was being courted by one of my paternal uncles(grand uncle) who later became the chief of the town of Bulbia.

The Bulbi- Naa (the chief of Bulbia) at the time desired to marry my grandmother, but she vehemently declined, and that began a whole series of retaliation. The chief wanted to punish my stubborn grandmother in some way. "Who is she to refuse my marriage proposal?" said the chief. "She is not going to take my brother's children back to her village Prima," reiterated the chief. The chief wanted to punish my grandmother, Tiyasi, in some painful way, but he could not think of any, thought my grandmother.

He wanted whatever he did to be so painful as to get my grandmother to have a change in her desire and love for him.

My grandmother did not seem to know who he was dealing with because nobody ever defied the courtship of the chief. The chief decided to take any action that would be so well publicized, affect my grandmother emotionally immensely and make her to change her mind.

Lo and behold, there came a British General (representing the British colonizers). The General at that time was scavenging for potential good children to go to school. He had made several trips to my village without any success. In most cases, children who had no parents or who were children of slaves were sent to the colonial schools.

The British representative also came to the village to collect taxes from the chief of the village or his designated representative. Most of the taxes collected were from cattle ownership by the farmers in the village. He also often scavenged for potential good children to go to school in the the Northern territories. He had made several unsuccessful trips to get children who could be trained the British way and come back to help effect rule on the natives. In most cases, the chosen children either had no parents or were children of slaves (Daaba)..

After a long discussion as to what they wanted or expected, my step-granduncle decided that he had to send one of my grandmother's children to school with the British representative. At this point in time, the chief almost always chose the child of a slave since it was considered a punishment to both the child and the mother. The system was not interested in educating girls, and my grandmother did not have any to offer.

My senior father, who was older, was deemed too old to go to school. He was not the one my granduncle was after the most to put a dagger into my grandmother's heart. My uncle was already farming and it was also a good enough reason not to send him to school. It was then decided that my father was the most reasonable alternative. My father was younger, had no experience working on the farm and was much closer to grandma Tiyasi. My granduncle also felt that my father would be a better ambassador representing the village, the Kantonsi tribe, the Mamprusi tribal owners, and the Northern territories of Ghana at large even though it was not his main reason for wanting to send my daddy to school..

Education at this time was mainly obtained by children of slaves because of the hardships the children and family had to go through. It involved long-distance walking barefooted, staying away for long periods of time during the year, and, in some cases, bullying in and out of school.

The slave owners did not want their children to go through these problems or hardships.

All along, it was known that the chief wanted to find a way to get my grandmother to marry him; and since she refused, he was ready to pay my grandmother back.

On one cool night grand-uncle (the chief) came into my grandmother's compound to announce to her that he had chosen her younger son to be sent far away for school.

There was no long discussion, and my grandmother's opinion did not matter, but she was full of grief and annoyance.

My father was prepared hastily and left the village with the British representative. He was sent to Gambaga Primary School and eventually ended up in Tamale for his middle school education. My grandmother wept cold tears for several weeks after her youngest son was sent several miles away from her. She would never understand the fact that her younger son was taken away from her.

She went deeper and deeper into a shell, according to my maternal grandmother. She kept to herself and never spoke to my granduncle until she died.

She began to turn around when my father occasionally came home on vacations and looked well. It took him three years before my grandmother saw him on his first vacation.

Travel was very difficult in those days.. There were no paved roads, and he had to walk for three to four days from school to get home through narrow winding paths and thick forest infested by kangaroos and snakes.

After the middle school education, he then went into Achimota Teachers Training College in Accra, the capital city of Ghana. It was an agony to go through according to my father. He barely returned to the village because he was now about four hundred miles away from home and could not readily get home or get money to travel at will. He was often sent home on vacation by the Regional British Council whenever the school could transport them home. At this time vehicles were very rare, and one could walk the four hundred miles or could purchase a horse or donkey to ride home if one could afford it. No formidable road system existed then. When there was an earthquake in Accra that killed a lot of people, 'my grandmother was heard walling about her son. My father had a cut across his face when part of his dormitory roof in Achimota Teachers Training college collapsed during the earthquake in Accra.

After about ten years when my father had left home, his brother died, and my grandmother was lonelier than ever, and she did not hide her feelings to the chief. To add to her misery my father could not attend his own brother's funeral because he was in school.

After the training college education was over, my father then started to teach in the primary and middle schools in the then Northern Region of Ghana. After his training, my father came back triumphantly.

My father did suffer as my grandmother expected because he often had to walk barefooted to school over several miles and often took several days of walking. He barely had any extra money to spend since my grandparents were subsistence farmers and was very poor.

He loved school and enjoyed going to school, which made life easier for my grandmother.

After his return from his schooling, my grandmother had picked the most beautiful girl she thought would be good for my father and bring him happiness. This wonderful woman she chose was to be later my mother and my saving grace.

When my father started teaching, he was often transferred from one school to the next to open new schools in the northern territories of the country.

As children, we never stayed in one town for an extended period of time.

My father opened and taught in new schools including Sandema, Zuarangu, Binduri, Nalerigu, Walewale, and numerous others in the northern territories of Ghana. My father was the first head teacher of the Walewale Middle Boarding School now called Walewale Secondary Technical School. I can barely remember the opening day of the school and the singing of the school's anthem, which was written by my father in Mampruli. My older sisters can still remember the words to the anthem. At a recent visit to the school, which I later attended as a student, the headmaster of the school did not even know anything about the history of the institution that he was now leading.

He taught school for about thirty-five years and eventually resigned. According to narratives, my grandmother became happier after she saw her son being educated and making money, and she became the envy of the village and surrounding villages.

My uncles, who were from favorite wives, became very jealous when they found that my father was making a teacher's salary and taking very good care of his beloved mother. She was noted to sing songs in Mampruli thanking my granduncle for trying to hurt her but instead he helped her. She thought that if my granduncle were alive to see her son, he would have regretted sending him to school to spite her.

We the children often looked back and laughed about it that it was because of our stubborn and opinionated grandmother who had defied all rules of tradition and religion and the role of the woman in society then that led us to become educated, and the whole Yamusah clan are forever grateful to our grandmother Tiyasi for the sacrifices she made that led to our father being sent to school.

My grandmother was alive to see her son have the first six children when she passed away peacefully.

My father cried like a baby when she died according to my mother, and it showed the whole family how much love he had for his mother and what she had gone through for him.

Father's Retirement from Teaching and return to the village, Bulbia as a farmer.

After my father resigned as a head teacher in 1963, he did not stay in Walewale, but we went to stay with his maternal cousin in the village of Wungu. Wungu is the traditional capital of the West Mamprusi District in Ghana. The Wungu-Naa is the traditional chief of villages west of Walewale, which is the political capital of the now West Mamprusi District Administration.

My father's cousin virtually had to move from his compound to give my father and the entire family his building—a series of mud huts. The children at this point then started going to Wungu Primary School. My oldest sister, Azuma, had already completed her Nursing Assistant training at the Nalerigu Baptist Medical Centre while my second oldest sister Sala, was also just starting her secondary school in Navrongo Secondary School (NAVASCO). My oldest brother, Yidana had already completed his Secondary School training at Asamankese Secondary School in Southern Ghana and was now a middle school teacher. The year I started middle school was the year my father decided to move back to his ancestral home in Bulbia. My father took up farming as a hobby and also worked to feed the family.

As school time was getting nearer, he had to make up his mind on what he wanted to do with all the children. He decided to send us to the Middle Boarding School, which was about fifteen miles away but felt as if it was more than a hundred-mile journey since we had to walk the distance barefooted whenever we were going to school at the beginning of the semester (term) or at the end of the term.

At this time vehicles were not readily available, and lorries and other vehicles were only available if we had money on Bulbia market days. The market day was and still only once a week, and a lot of trading went on including buying and selling of items produced on our local farms. On market days my mother did a lot of trading selling fish and *kenkey* (corn dough).

On holidays we often would "help" my mother in the market. She also always made us have lunch in her market stall.

One day a woman came into our stall to buy some kenkey. She saw us eating, and she was surprised. She asked my mother why she was feeding us from the same food she was making to sell to the public. After several minutes of looking at us eat, she concluded that my mother's food's quality had to be good if she was feeding her own children with the same food she was selling to the public. This woman was like a one-person advertisement. My mother's stall was often full as word went across the market and village. My mother worked hard to get us to school. She did every job that she could get her hands on in order to purchase food and household items we needed. She often walked to Bimbini to buy fresh fish to sell. She will often get up at four o'clock in the morning to pick Shea butter nuts to sell so that we could get monies to go back to school. What did my mother not do to keep the family going after my father resigned from teaching?

At the time also some of my uncle's children who were staying with my father whilst going to school decided that it was too much for them to walk the distance and did not want to stay in boarding schools. About three of my cousins dropped out from school. There was intense pressure from my uncles to my father to stop my sisters from going to school. My uncles were Muslims and traditionalists and did not believe in educating girls because they believed that the girls were going to be morally indoctrinated or become prostitutes because of Western influence. My father, however, refused and insisted that we all had to go to Walewale to attend the boarding school.

This was the beginning of some intense trials and errors. We would wake up around four o'clock in the morning and initiate walking, carry luggage on our heads, and make several stops along the road to eat. Most of this walk was done barefooted and we were often accompanied by my mother or step mother to make sure we got to school safely.

My mother never had any formal education. In those days my grandparents were traditionalists, and even though they did not practice Islam, our Kantonsi tradition was similar in the sense of not educating females.

My mother, however, had started trading and going to the White Volta River near our village to buy and sell fish. My maternal grandmother prepared my mother to become prepared as a teacher's wife and the demands that came with it.

According to my maternal grandmother, other families were also grooming their daughters for my father too; but when he came back after his education, he decided to marry my mother, and the rest is history. My mother continued to trade. She sold kenkey (corn), fish, and often rice and beans (*sinkafa da waché*). This trade would end up sending all the children to school since my father's teacher's salary was very small and not enough for a large family like ours.

I am one out of nine children from my mother's side. My junior mother or stepmother Adisah had six children, mother Aduku had two children and Mother Samata whom I did not have an opportunity to meet had also two children before she left our household.. We were a very close family in a polygamous setting, and to show the respect I had for my stepmother, Adisa, I have named one of my children after her.

Growing up Crippled:
The role my mother, family, herbalism, Mbazoa and religion plays in my recovery from being Crippled.

As a child, I was unique in some ways. I tended to do things late developmentally and also was afflicted by all childhood diseases known at that time.

The most serious problem I went through was my inability to walk. My younger brother who was born about eleven months after me grew up and was able to walk, run, and do things faster than I did. In today's world I would have been considered autistic. I even had to be carried to school the first few years by my father because of my inability to walk. No reasons could be given to explain why I could not walk. I was considered a' Gbariga' (a person who is disabled and cannot walk. There were speculations that my ancestors had angered our Bulbia deities to the accusation that some how I was sacrificed for witchcraft and finally the work of the devil is a common blame in African society. My siblings were very mean since they knew I could not walk or run after them.

They would come and purposely step on me and run away. As soon as I screamed, which I perfected, my mother would come out screaming and wanting to find out who it was who intentionally stepped on me or hit me and ran away.

It was usually my older sister Sala who seemed to get a kick out of hearing me scream.

All my siblings thought that my mother was paying too much attention to me and not to them.

I did all I could to remedy this situation, but my legs could not carry the rest of my body. When I was born, I had multiple infections as a baby, and my mother could count the number of days I felt well.

I was diagnosed from having malaria and all sorts of witchcraft to the possession of the devil in me. My mother, in trying to remedy my situation, carried me to all variations of medicine that were available and accessible in Northern Ghana.

My first encounter with modern medicine was when I developed an inguinal infection, which had to be excised and drained. At the age of about six, which I can still remember vividly today, my mother made sure I did not forget it. It was the first time that any of my family members had been admitted to Nalerigu Baptist Medical Center in Nalerigu, Northern Region, Ghana.

At about three to four years of age, when every boy or girl is expected to stop breast feeding it seemed that I rather perfected it and continued to breastfeed even though my younger brother had stopped.

I was generally ill looking, and my siblings thought that I was pretending not to be able to walk for sympathy and to get my mother's attention. They all thought I was selfish. What they did not know was that I hated the position metted me and I did everything a child could do to defend myself.

After some of these infections, I had running nose and diarrhea. I could not use my lower extremity to ambulate or stand even more.. .

My mother became very frantic and wanted to find out what it was that made my legs so weak that they could not hold me up.

After several visits to the Baptist Medical Center and other government hospitals, my mother decided to send me to an Imam who was also my father's friend who was known to cure all kinds of diseases. He was also a known natural healer (*warizam*) in the community.

All along my mother had done research of all the known fetish priests and traditional medical experts, but none could help her suffering son. I did not realize that it was taking a toll on my mother and the rest of the family.

As it was customary in those days and still today in Ghana and numerous African countries, if you were crippled, you were considered a devil, a curse to your family and society at large, and considered as punishment to a family for past bad deeds that were committed by one's ancestors; and one was often chastised and vilified in society. Most crippled people were eventually thrown out on the streets and became beggars as is common up to today in most Ghanaian societies. People would often throw things at you and equate you to the working of the devil.

My mother was determined not to do that to her son, and she took the blame that somehow it was her fault that I was crippled and bore all the social pressure to take care of her crippled son..

One day after discussions with my father and some maternal uncles, my mother packed our belongings, and we were on our way to Gambaga. My siblings were left with Mother Adisah because my mother was confident they would all be taken care of well by her.

My mother tied me up in the back and walked with me to the lorry station, and eventually we got a lorry and ended up in Mbazoa's (my father's friend) house. She had made arrangement so that we could stay with Mbazoa's oldest wife in her hut (Duu). My mother helped with the daily chores whilst I began what she hoped would end up getting me to walk.

Every morning I would crawl in front of the imam's prayer area with my mother, and prayers were said over me.

Pouring libation and animal sacrifices were also made to my ancestors in case family members living or dead had done something wrong to infuriate my ancestors. Mbazoa tried to straighten my legs, but they were so weak. He held me and told me to support him by holding on to him. I just had no power in my legs, and they immediately would become flaccid and make me flop down. I remember these events as if it was today because I went through a very painful yet challenging period of my life, which has made me to be able to withstand major stress in my lifetime.

Mbazoa kept rubbing my legs with a solution from a talisman and also from some grounded roots. My feet would burn, and my muscle would twitch and itch at the same time.

He kept separating my legs and binding them at the knees and other portions of my lower extremity.

I should have guessed that something dramatic was about to happen.

On one Friday when people would donate food to the poor and needy this particular day, there was a big crowd outside and inside the compound drumming and singing local songs and dancing. My mother was summoned to Mbazoa's compound and his teaching center where he taught Arabic and also thought other Islamic converts about Koranic teachings.

My mother was made to sit me near her lap, and as usual, I could hear my mother praying to anyone who would listen and answer her prayer.

Suddenly a middle-aged man appeared with a white hat and a long white robe holding a very big hen. The hen was tied at its legs and laid in front of me. I started to play with the hen. My mother quickly pulled my hands away and told me to pay attention to what was happening.

The drumming and songs grew closer and closer and also louder and louder.

Another group of Mankaranta students (religious students) in the same robes joined our group. My mother was the only female present in this ceremony. Mbazoa started to recant some words that he had written in a slate (wooden talisman) in front of him.

After he finished recanting these words, he looked up to my mother. My mother showed an anguish in her face but was ready for anything that would help get his son to walk.

He then took four sticks separated by what I thought was mud and laid them in front of me.

He asked my mother to put me close to him.

Again whilst Mbazoa was enchanting his program, he rapped those flat wooden sticks to each of the hen's legs and laid it at the corner of his praying room.

The sticks were well molded with mud. As much I can remember at the age of five or six and from my mother, the hen did not make much noise, but obviously my mother by the look of her face was touched by the cracking of the legs of the hen.

After molding the arranged sticks with mud, he again started his enchantment or prayers, and then a period of absolute silence followed.

The atmosphere was very peaceful, and the hen was not moving from place to place. Mbazoa then asked my mother if she believed in him and what he was doing. "Do you believe Allah can make miracles?" he asked my mother.

My mother who was now kneeling in prayer emphatically said yes and indicated that if she did not believe in him and Allah she would not bring her problems to him and Allah and our ancestors to help her solve them.

He lifted my hands up and asked my mother to straighten my legs up and said to my mother, "The day the hen stands to walk will be the day your son will also walk."

After he dropped my hands, I held on to my mother very tightly because a breeze of fear had come into me. He then asked my mother to take some break to our hut where we were staying with his oldest wife.

My mother assisted his oldest wife to go to the well to fetch water and go to the market to buy food for us on market days. In the mornings my mother would allow me to crawl to a baobab tree in front of the house to play with other kids in the neighborhood who were not any different from my own siblings because I was insulted and called a cripple and other undesirable names by these kids. They were even meaner than my own siblings.

Unlike when I cried when my siblings would call me such names and harass me because of my disability to walk, I did not cry to these hideous kids. I instead told them to get close to me if they were brave enough. I also kept telling them that I would soon be able to walk and catch up with them.

One of Mbazoa's sons would come and exercise my feet by stretching and rubbing an ointment, which was highly scented, on my feet. I was not in pain and began to feel some strength and vibrations down my legs. Several weeks passed by that I forgot all about the chicken, which had its legs broken, and the wooden molds placed since there were many hens running around most of the day in the compound. Amazingly my mother never said anything about them but seemed very nervous and was not herself. I, however, began to feel some tingling in my legs; but more startling, I began to get some pains and feelings I did not experience before.

At about six to eight weeks after we had gone through the ritual of breaking the hen's legs, my mother was summoned to the prayer room where the chicken was kept and taken care of.

It was just after the morning prayers. She came and packed me up and brought me into the designated room.

Mbazoa came in with his familiar dignified and elegant pose and sat a distance from my mother and myself. This time he also had some assistants with him who were Junior imams learning the Koran from him. He began by praying, and after the prayers, he asked for the bound hen to be brought in. He again prayed when the hen was brought in, and this time the hen was laid on my lap. I resisted, but my mother held onto me as I began crying..

He began to dig out the mud around the sticks he placed on both legs of the hen and continuously looked into my face. He kept enchanting to himself because I could not hear a thing out of what he was saying. All the mud was gradually removed except the flat, well-trimmed, and aligned sticks. He asked my mother to straighten both my legs and to hold them straight and not to let them go even if I was in pain.

For the first time, I could not feel any resistance from my muscles or pains to the thighs. He again looked into my face and began to unwrap the rest of the sticks on the hen's legs, which were joined together by strings like a fence. During this whole period, he asked my mother to recite certain Koranic verses to his hearing. He completely unwrapped both legs. All this time the hen was on my legs held down by one of his assistants. The hen looked as helpless as I was. He told my mother if she was ready for what was to happen. "If the hen stands up and walks and does not fall back to the ground, your son will also do the same," said Mbazoa. "Do you have the faith that Allah and your ancestors will allow this to happen?" Mbazoa asked. "Yes," said my mother. He clapped both hands together and made a loud noise with both bands. His assistant let the wings of the hen go, and suddenly the chicken was up. It looked around as if it was looking for me and began to slowly walk out. Mbazoa started to smile, and all I could hear was "Allahu Kubaru, Allahu Kubaru" said several times. He told my mother to stand up. I looked at him and thought that the man was possibly getting crazy. He was shivering, and my mother let me go with no hesitation as if she was commanded to. After my mother let me go for the first time in my life, I could feel the weight of my body on my legs. Suddenly the hen with no guidance from anybody as much as I could see passed between my legs, and as if the ground began to move, I felt myself moving, and my mother held on to me. Mbazoa said to my mother, "Let him go in the name of Allah." Without hesitation my mother let me go. Suddenly I was alone taking two steps. My feet felt very heavy, but they were moving.

"*Mma* [my mother] Mma, Mma, I can walk," I shouted. My mother tried to embrace me, but the assistant refused. I took three or four steps unsturdingly and thought that I was going to fall, but I kept going. All along Mbazoa kept his enchantment and salutations going, and his voice began to intensify. As if there was no gravity, I began to walk, and the hen continued to flap its wings between my legs.

After a couple more steps, Mbazoa asked my mother to put me back on her lap again. One of his assistants came toward me and started rubbing my legs with an ointment and a very cold peppermint-scented mud-like material. My legs suddenly felt heavier, and my mother after some words from Mbazoa was asked to take me back to my hut. The hen was left free. I could identify the hen no matter how many hens were in the compound at the same time. Every morning Mbazoa's assistant would come to the hut we were staying in and rub my legs with the same ingredients. He would also walk with me and did exercises in my legs. I was eventually given a pulley-like walker to use at all times.

One day, as I was walking, I fell down, and my mother came running and crying thinking I was injured; but before she could get to me, I had started to get up by myself and walked toward her. This was the first time I could see the joy and happiness and almost a relief of pressure from the nature of her smile to me. She suddenly started sobbing as if somebody had died. To me at that point, my mother was saying that all the pressure she had undergone had a fruitful ending.

My mother walked briskly to Mbazoa's compound and was still crying.

With the aid of the imam's assistants, I found my mother again on the floor sobbing but thanking Mbazoa for all he did. He turned around and looked at me and said, "It's your mother's faith in Allah and me that has brought you to this point." I could not stand seeing my mother crying so much so I laid on top of her back and started to sob in joy too with my mother.

"Take your son and get some rest," said Mbazoa. "We still have more work to do," he added. He had not yet given my mother any permission to go back to Nalerigu. We had spent about six months in Gambaga and had left the rest of my siblings and father behind with my stepmother, Adisah. I could see the resentment my siblings had against me because they felt that I was getting all the attention, which they also needed.

My daily chores, walking and being massaged in the legs, continued. Because of our long absence, my father had decided to come to see us. My father, who was not a man of many words, was shocked to see me playing outside the compound. He had seen me outside the compound in front of the big baobab tree but did not recognize me because he did not expect me to be standing. He actually walked past my group without seeing me, and I had not seen him too.

He went into the compound. He took off his shoes as it is customary and after speaking to my mother came back looking for me. He came back to the tree to make sure it was his son and then went into the compound to greet his friend. I was not allowed into or near the exchange between my father and Mbazoa.

My father came out to leave. He was told by my mother not to tell anybody in the house, neighborhood, or the town of Nalerigu about what she described as a miracle until she brought me home. After speaking with my mother, he came to the tree and picked me up as if to say, "Is this real?" I definitely liked that, and after about a two-hour visit, he left to go back to the rest of the family. My therapy continued for another two weeks.

One Friday before prayers, Mbazoa's summoned my mother who was still in shock to let my mother know that it was not he who relieved me of my ailment but that it was again the work of Allah and my mother's faith in his ability to work with Allah. Mbazoa told my mother that she could prepare to take me home within a week. I continued to work at the beginning with sincere fear of falling, but I never did after the above referenced episode. My mother watched me even more carefully and did not go to the market or to fetch water at the well as often as before when I started to walk without taking me along even though I was not the youngest sibling at the time. I gained more confidence as the time went by, and my mother gradually got more confident that her prayers were truly answered through the powers of Allah and her ancestors. Since then my mother has remained a very devout Muslim and hardly misses praying five times a day until Allah called her home on the twenty-fourth of March, 2012. The basic religion of the Kantonsi tribe to which I belong is Islam. My mother often took me to prayers especially on Friday evenings. Since women always prayed at the back of the male congregation, I was always in the back with my mother.

One Friday before evening prayers, my mother was summoned to the mosque by the imams of the village. The evening prayers were said, and after the prayers, the imam asked my mother and me to the front. All of a sudden, there was a loud applause among the congregation. As if embarrassed, I ran back to hold on to my mother tightly. I looked into my mother's eyes, and she was crying again.

We were released to return to Nalerigu by Mbazoa on Monday. My mother got up very early in the morning and washed me up and cleaned everything we had brought with us. She also made porridge for breakfast. She knelt before Mbazoa's senior wife and thanked her for her goodwill and help in accommodating us. She then parked our meager belongings, and we went into Mbazoa's compound.

As a custom, my mother would often take her shoes off her feet before going to a mosque to see Mbazoa. It was a sign of meekness and respect. Also, she never looked directly into Mbazoa's eyes. She knelt alone and held me out. Mbazoa asked her to let me come to him, and I did. He gave me a talisman to wear around my waist and a wrist talisman for me to keep. He tossed me up in the air as if to make sure my legs were present and placed me back down. My mother again could not stop crying and sobbing. At least this time it was for joy, happiness, and disbelief of what she called a miracle rather than from frustration.

Mbazoa thanked Allah and our ancestors and said a prayer by putting his right hand on my forehead and then authorized my mother to take me home. "Make sure you do not lose these talismans, my son," said Mbazoa, "and great things will come out of you."

My mother got up slowly, genuflected toward Mbazoa, held my hand, and we left Mbazoa's compounds. "Words cannot express the gratitude I owe to this man," said my mother. "It is only Allah or God who can repay him."

We went out, took our belongings, and said goodbye to Mbazoa's other wives and children and left for the lorry station in Gambaga to get a ride back home. The lorry took off after about two and a half hours, and my mother would not let me go. She held on to me very tightly as if to say she did not want to risk any misfortune.

The lorry arrived in Nalerigu market and lorry station late in the evening. Nobody in my family anticipated our return home, and as such, no one was at the lorry station to meet us. We had to walk about a mile to get home. My mother insisted on still carrying me on her back as if she did not want me to take a chance harming what Allah had just fixed. She had her luggage on her head, and I was propped up in the back as big as I was. She walked briskly and sang songs of praise to Allah and our ancestors along the whole route home. When she approached our bungalow, she untied her cloth that held me on her back and brought me down to walk. It was the slowest time I had ever noticed my mother take to set me down from her back onto the ground to walk. She was extra cautious. All of a sudden, my father who had gone for his usual evening walk and was now about to sit on his lazy chair saw us. He walked toward us and as if he did not see us sat back down. He got up a second time and looked. At this time he started running toward us. This was the first time I ever saw my father running outside a tennis court. He got to me first because my mother had me walking in front. He picked me up, and for the first time in my life, I saw my father sobbing. When I saw tears flow down my father's face, it shocked me because I did not think that he felt the same pain and pressure as my mother did. He picked me up, gave me a squeeze, and laughed after the tears. My mother as soon as she saw her husband in tears started to sob in joy. "Can you see your son walking?" asked my mother to my father.

"Your friend and Allah have performed wonders, and my son is now walking," she screamed. "Contrary to people telling me that my son should be thrown away because he was crippled, Allah to whom all things are possible has relieved us of all the shame and anguish," she added.

He walked patiently with his back to the house and asked me to wait outside. In the house my mother and father went in first and asked me to wait outside. She had to go through her rituals, which were routinely carried out whenever a family member returned from a trip. I still have to undergo it whenever I visit home, even though I lost my mother at about the age of ninety-five in 2012. There was a big applause. I heard my older sister ask my mother where her crippled son was. My mother, as if not to acknowledge her, called me to come in. All my siblings stood quietly when they saw me walking for the first time in their presence. They all came up and embraced me, and almost in unison, Mother Adisah and my siblings all started to cry. They could not help holding their mother because they had not seen her in over six months.

She had put everything aside including the care of her other children for her crippled son. It was then that I realized that my sister and brothers resented that my mother had put her effort on one child and that, in turn, they resented me by stepping on me and running. No more, no more stepping on me and running, because I can run to get you, even though I was still limited to the distance I could run. Besides, my mother would not allow me to run. My mother no longer had to shout at the top of her voice to protect her crippled son, and she could stop training for the Olympics in order to catch up with my siblings and neighborhood bullies who could step on me and run only to be chased down by my mother.

Walking meant a lot to me personally because it meant that I could protect myself, I could go to school without being carried, and I did not have to be stared at like an alien object. Walking relieved me of all negative name calling, but most important of all, it resolved my parents of feeling guilty that they or their ancestors had been punished for wrongdoing or ill will, which in Ghanaian and African culture still plays an important role. Any disability or developmental deformity is considered a curse from the Almighty or our ancestors. Walking meant a lot, but I also continued to be cautious and had my limitations. Walking meant that I could defend myself in school. Importantly I could go to school during the day and attend Makaranta (Koranic) lessons at night. I did not have to be carried to school by my father to the stare of the world. I could not initially walk as fast as my other siblings or friends out of fear of falling, but the more walking I did without falling, the more confident I became.

I became interested in Islam and went into a Makaranta school (evening Koranic learning school) to learn the Arabic necessary to read the Holy Koran. I went to a Western-style education in the daytime and to an Islamic school at night.

In both schools I stayed focused in my education. I did not have to be carried to school. I did not have to be settled in one place, and most of all I did not have to be called derogatory names. Most Ghanaian disabled children often do not have the mother and father to give the care they gave me. My mother, as well as Mother Adisah, sacrificed, and my father and all my siblings extended themselves to help me even though my siblings could be as mean as the street. I did spring up from being disabled to become one who could work and function. As a result, I did not end up on the streets begging to make a living since most of the disabled at the time did and still live on the streets and lorry parks in Ghana, most of Africa, and every other country in this world.

I found out that I became more interested in school because I could challenge my older and younger sibling and classmates to certain subjects they did not know or did not wish to learn. School was also a place l felt confident and indeed became a source of help to the same people who thought I was nobody. Hence, I became a tutor at my early years for non-intelligent but rich kids.

I often taught them or helped them with their homework. In turn they brought bread, biscuits, and pastries that were not available to me. I often parked them up and carried them home to share with my sibling. I also made some money, which I used to buy books and made my own library and shared them with my siblings and friends.

In most societies in those days, children from rich homes were generally not smart and did not have to work hard to survive, so they had no incentive to study to succeed in life.

Being from a relatively poor family depending on a teacher's salary, I wanted to get off poverty and often thought that through education I could get myself and my mother in particular out of poverty and build my parents a beautiful home.

I also used my good penmanship to assist students by copying their class notes, and in turn, I got paid for it. I was not allowed to play sports by my parents who still had an element of fear that something could happen to revert me back to where l was before.

Primary school education, school bullying and snake bite experience.

After my father's resignation from teaching in 1963 and just about that time my walking was now intact, I went to Walewale Middle School after completing my primary school education in Wungu, which is about twelve miles from my village Bulbia. I studied hard, but due to several factors, I was not one of the favorite students by my seniors. I was often excused from my eighth and ninth grade classes and taken to the senior classes by their class teacher to tutor them in mathematics and English. The seniors resented that their junior was chosen to teach them mathematics, English, and science. I was made to lash or whip them with a cane if they did not get the answers right. Since this was a boarding middle school, we lived on campus. At night the seniors would make up excuses in order to retaliate because of the lashing or whipping I was required to give them by their teacher. Whenever I was reluctant to do the caning, the teacher would often show me the best way to whip them by whipping me. This, in addition with the fact that they drummed up charges to punish me in boarding school, was enough incentive for me to learn how to hold the cane and whip well since they often retaliated at night in the most cruel of ways. The seniors would come over to my bedding at night, pour water onto my bed, and turn around and accuse me of wetting my bed at night.

Wetting the bed in a boarding school was a punishable offence, and even though they were intentionally drummed up by my dormitory prefect, I still got punished. After some time, I could not take the punishment anymore. I made up excuses in order not to have to teach my seniors in form four how to study mathematics. On some occasions they let me kneel on gravel in the middle of the dormitory until I began bleeding from my knees. Despite several complaints, the class teacher did not believe me that these atrocities were going on in the dormitory in the night. When confronted, the seniors would deny that such atrocities were going on, and every student in dormitory was afraid to tell the truth since such atrocities were being committed by my less intelligent seniors.

The headmaster Mr. Y who had taken over after my father resigned was an assistant to my father before he resigned. He did not like my father because he thought that my father was supposedly arrogant to him. He actually encouraged the seniors and prefects of the school to punish me even though I was the brightest student the school ever had and it ends up that I am the first and only student of the school to ever become a medical doctor.

On one occasion, I was locked up in the storage room, where they stored garden equipment and books, because of my refusal to tutor my upperclassmen. The truth was that because of all the punisment i was taking was unbearable; it was my desire to end my tutoring services that was forced on me that the student leaders left me in a hot, smelly and mosquito infested room. Left and locked in a dark, hot and foul smelling room overnight,. Looking for a place to escape; the back window wasnot fully locked ; so I lifted the window and crawled out of the dark room into the back of WaleWale Middle school that was bushy, full of trees and very wet.

In the thick darkness of the night and walking barefooted in a snake-infested area, I heard a hissing-like sound It was so dark that the ground could not be seen and apparently I had just stepped on what I thought was a snake which bit me in return. This ended my journey to my village. Running away to go to my village and report to my family what was going on in the boarding school was cut short.

My maternal uncle, Kpabinaba, who was a herbalist, had often preached to us what to do in case we suspected a snake bite. So as soon as I came in contact with what I thought and felt was a snake bite and seeing some moonlight shining as I got out of the thick bush, I immediately took a sharp rock, which was not hard to find, and cut across the upper part of my right leg where the pain was. I squeezed as hard as I could to get blood and the venom out. My maternal uncle, whom I accompanied to the bush to look for medicinal herbs, had taught me how to handle snake bites in case there was ever a suspicion of a snake bite. He even had illustrated it to us on one of our trips to find a medicinal herb called 'muhiri', which he used for migraine headaches. He reiterated that if one waited too long in deciding whether a bite was from a snake or not, it could mean living or dying. He often emphasized to err on treating such a bite as a snake bite and managing as such until proven otherwise. After letting as much blood out the upper part of my right leg, I made a rope out of a bush tree that was on the side of the Wungu road and tied it tightly around my right calf.

As the moon shown more, I walked listlessly to my maternal aunt's house, which was in downtown Walewale, and not to the health center, which was literally in front of me as I came down the hill. As soon as my aunt Lahari saw me, she asked me what I wanted in town this late at night. She started to chastise me, but when she was recounted my story of having been bitten by a snake. she hurriedly called her husband, and attention was sought for me. I was then placed in bed rest after I told my maternal aunt and her husband what I had done which was what my maternal uncle, the traditional doctor, had taught me to do if there was ever a suspicion of ever being bitten by a snake. I could not go to school the next day. The form four teacher who had authorized me to tutor his senior class that resulted in my running away from school had enquired and came to my aunt's house to find me.

All of a sudden, it dawned on me what I just did. I cut the same legs I have had problems walking with, and I immediately became scared and delirious that I was going to lose my legs. My maternal aunt's husband applauded me for what I did to save my own life, and I told him I had learnt it from my uncle in the village.

I was taken to Walewale clinic, which was not far from the boarding school, for checkup. The dispenser was called Mr. Azuri, who cleaned up the wound site and reinforced the new dressing and took my improvised bandage which consisted of leaves.

The next afternoon my aunt came running to me saying that my father had just arrived on his bicycle from the village and that news had already got to him about me being bitten by a snake. The school, seeing that I was missing in the storage room where I was locked up, sent somebody on a motorcycle to inform my parents of my absence from school. This day was a Walewale market day; and after within three hours, my mother, who had walked twelve miles, arrived later. I was pale and weak, but my father told me that I had taken the right remedies and was surprised I had been taught by my uncle.

My mother and father stayed with me in my aunt's house until I got better, and they then left for the village.

I had escaped death again, and after this incident, my aunt insisted I stay with her whilst going to school as a day scholar instead of going back to the boarding halls..

I jumped with joy because I was really scared to go back to school because of all the punishment that was being bestowed on me because my mathematics teacher encouraged me to whip seniors I was forced to tutor.

About two weeks after I went back to school in my second year of middle school education, I had to sit for the Ghana government common entrance examination, which was a standardized examination for all second-, third-, and fourth-year middle school students. Those who passed this examination went into a secondary school of their choice. I took this examination along with my brother, which later had its own consequences. As a day scholar, I was recruited to teach English in the Walewale adult night school to the illiterate parents, store owners, and other business people in the town of WaleWale.. A lot of the night school students were motivated, and I also made some money to buy myself new books and a spare school uniform. Late at night after teaching in the night school ; I then went to sell tea in the WaleWale lorry station. It was considered demeaning for a student to work at a public place like a tea shop, but to me I did not consider it in any way demeaning as long I was being paid and I did not have to depend solely on my poor parents for everything I needed or wanted.

I worked for about four hours at night during the week and about eight hours on the weekends. It did not affect my grades in school.

I used these monies to buy my review study guides and other essentials, and I often shared my money and review books with my younger brother who had come to live with me at our aunt's house. My brother needed a lot of things, but he was not eager to work as I did. He, however, borrowed my books, and he knew he could depend on me to help him up anytime the need arose. The owner of the tea shop was also one of my adult night school students. After about two months, I was called to the headmaster's office and told that I had passed the common entrance examination to my first choice, Navrongo Secondary School, and also Notre Dame Secondary in the same town, which was about seventy miles away from my village. My brother also passed and had to go to Bawku Secondary School. We were very few students in the Mamprusi District who had passed, and proudly both Yamusah's children had passed the National Common Entrance Examination. Instead of my headmaster Mr. Y being happy for us, it was distasteful when he called my brother and me to let us know that the local council was not going to sponsor both Yamusah's children since it had never happened in the district that two family members had passed the common entrance examination at the same time. The headmaster, however, told me that two students from the same household could not go on to secondary school at the same time under the Local Government scholarship.. This had never happened before according to the headmaster. The local council, which sponsored and paid for the secondary school fees, was informed that the Headmaster had decided not to sponsor me even though I had the second highest score in the whole of the Northern and Upper regions of Ghana at the time.

It was toward the end of the school term, so we went home and spoke to our parents about the predicament I was in. My father thought that it was a deliberate act by the headmaster to deny me scholarship when I had one of the best test scores in the whole country whilst the local council was sponsoring students from Nigeria, Burkina Faso (Upper Volta), and the Ivory Coast.

My mother Adisa called me into her hut and spoke to me and told me not to worry over issues ii had no control over, and she promised something very positive would come out of this experience. As it was customary, it was announced by the chief in the village and also to Grandmother Amina, whom I was very close to, and she wondered why I wanted go to school when I could get a job. "I see because your big head is empty of any brain," she often said jokingly. "That is why they want to keep you in school longer." After about a week, I went back to Walewale to work at the tea shop to help pay for my school uniform, some of the school fees, and travel expenses to Navrongo Secondary School.

SECOND PHASE OF ZARA'S CRIPPLED SON'S LIFE

Secondary school education in Navrongo Secondary School in Ghana.

N avrongo Secondary School located in the town of Navrongo now in the Upper East Region of Ghana was the school I most wanted to attend for my secondary school education. The two main reasons I most wanted to attend the school was because my older sister, Sala, was already enrolled there and was in her last year of her education and secondarily because the academic atmosphere in Navasco was a miniscule at that time even though Navsco had a good sports reputation in football and field hockey. The standardized G.C.E. 'O' level examination results for the first three years was not impressive at all. By going to Navasco I felt some contribution could be made by me to bolster the academic credentials of the school. Most of the bright Northern students with very good Commom Entrance Examination results were often recruited by the then academic powerhouses such as Bishop Herman Secondary School, Adisadel College, Prempeh College Mfanstpim college and Achimota School. At the secondary school level they also siphoned the students with the best 'O' level results to undertake their sixth form education, The Northern schools were then left with the not so bright Northern students and the southern mediocre students who had no other choice but to attend schools like Navasco Whatever was to be done on my behalf to contribute to reducing or eliminating this brain drain was a strong feeling that I had could be done by creating a competitive academic environment.

In about August 1966 I left for Navasco. When I got there, my sister was ending her secondary school education. The first-year students to secondary school commonly called' Green Leaves' had to go through an initiation period. On the first day of opening of my first term in Navasco, as soon as we arrived on campus, the initiation period to the school started. We the Green Leaves were made to carry our *potomanto* (luggage) from one dormitory to the other without being told which one we were to be housed in. We were made *to* carry on this routine till we became tired or until we virtually collapsed because of fatigue. We were eventually assigned to our dormitories, and the rest of the initiation took place in the night. The upperclassmen were responsible for these events of our initiation rites. My sister's presence in the school did not help since the boys' dormitories were completely different and far from the girls' dormitories.

Navasco had about a thousand boys and about thirty-five girls at the time.

When the initiation period began to look more like torture, my sister appeared from nowhere to tell her fellow students that I was her junior brother and how fragile I was.

The headmaster also had heard about the initiation period and was concerned about it. The headmaster came up and saved us from going through the whole process. My sister was very concerned especially about me carrying my luggage on my head and walking on a large school ground. The headmaster was seen speaking to my sister who later told me that she had expressed her concerns to the headmaster who indicated that I might have had a history of being handicapped but that i had no handicapped brains and that the school was very proud to have me choosing to come to his school. The headmaster was a red-haired Scottish man with an ulcerated saddle nose who was very hardworking and very nice. His name was Mr. Ramsey who dedicated himself to see a better Navasco.

I continued to study hard; and my strong subjects were English, German, mathematics, and chemistry. I did very well. I mainly remained to myself and liked to be alone. Some of my schoolmates thought that I was too eccentric, but to me it was a way to stay focused and worked hard to win a Cocoa Marketing Board Scholarship since my own local council would not sponsor my brother and me at the same time. My family had decided my brother was to get the scholarship. I was more than sure I was going to win an academic scholarship. I often walked to the school pond and garden area to study during the evenings after classes. The school pond was a place I could relax, pray, and pour my libation to my ancestors in peace.

I often studied at night, but due to shortage of energy products, all our school electricity was shut off about ten O'Clock at night. I sometimes used a candle to study. I did not have much or want a very involved social life in secondary school and was often called a bookworm which is the equivalent o a nerd today. I was a very shy young student who had an ambition to be a superb student and focused on why I had chosen to study in Navasco instead of going to schools down Southern Ghana that had far much better academic records than Navasco. I did not qualify to have a girlfriend because we only had thirty-five girls in the whole school, and one had to be either very good-looking or come from a popular and rich household. I did not qualify for any of these entities that often led one to land a girlfriend and frankly I felt I was too young and ambitious to involve myself in love affairs..

My religious teaching and background began to sway. I began to ask questions about religion, and in some cases nobody could give me a comprehensible or what I thought was an intelligent answer to my religious questions. One of the biggest concerns I had was why Arabic was not taught so that we could use it to communicate and write but only to read and recite the Koran. It was so much memorization that I can still recite some of the verses from the Koran in Arabic. For a person who was curious to learn and understand, there was often the question why I could not be taught to use the Arabic language if I went to the Sudan or Mali, which are areas of my descendants and also areas where Arabic is used in all facets of life.

Also, the amount of discipline was brutal and often involved whipping, and we often would shout louder to be heard even though we did not understand much of what we were reciting or being taught in Arabic. When I got into secondary school mainly because of my being able to read and understand Christianity, I started to drift in that direction. I never could discuss with my mother about some of my concerns in Islam. She had no explanations to some of my questions, which I understood. I often wondered why I could not worship and pray in both religious entities. In Christianity it seemed one had to confess and devote oneself to the Christian faith and teachings where one was taught that non-Christians would go to hell when they died. I could not reason with that because my beloved mother who had sacrificed for me at my tender age was not going to go to hell. I could not even lose faith in a religion that I definitely attributed saving my life up to today. My mother's religion and Mbazoa's belief and religion had brought me to this point in time, and I was very grateful and would not dare to disrespect it. On the other hand, here was a new religion, Christianity, which challenged my intellectual curiosity and could be understood by reading books, which I loved to do.

In Walewale, I had some friends who belonged to the Assemblies of God Church, which did not appeal to me. In secondary school I began to go to the Catholic church and found its solitude and teaching understanding and challenging. There were some aspect of Christianity that I questioned, but I figured it was like everything else in life. I began to figure it out that one cannot be hundred percent satisfied with all aspects of religious practices and faith. I read deeper and deeper about Christianity, and I felt a certain kind of peace in my mind that I felt I could belong to the teachings of Christ even though I could not understand all aspects of the Christian faith either.

A Catholic priest by the name of Father John had just been posted to Navasco, and he contributed to my choice of the Catholic faith. He was a Ghanaian priest with class and dignity. He had some simplicity to him, which I admired and respected. I had several conversations ongoing with him, and he also had an organized Christian teaching time, which enabled me to understand the religion. I continued to find myself going to church and eventually became baptized in school as a Christian.

Over the secondary school, I became the main Catholic student representative in the school and eventually became the first chaplain school prefect in Navasco's history.

When I went home, I discussed my newfound faith with my parents especially my mother, and she said that religion was an independent choice. She told me she had married my father despite the fact that my father was a pagan because she loved and respected him. She indicated to me that religion was a personal choice, and even though she wished I stayed a Moslem, she was not in any way annoyed with me.

"As you see, your father pours his libation, and I respect his religious view and participate willingly in it even though I was born and practice the Moslem faith. All you need is to respect all religions and the people who represent those religions," said my mother. They all have the same final goal.

She indicated that all religions have a mediator because nobody is powerful enough to pray directly to Allah or God. "Your father and traditional African religion believe that their ancestors take their messages to God, but Christians and Moslems believe in that Christ and Prophet Mohammed are the mediators to God. All religions are the same," said my mother.

I came out after this discussion feeling very good because I sincerely thought that my mother was going to object to it considering all the things she had gone through. All you need to do is to respect, love, and care for people because that is what religion is all about. I followed this principle until I became the chaplain prefect where I represented all religions not only the Christian faith alone.

In school all Christian and Moslem holidays were honored, and as chaplain prefect, I coordinated all religious activities in Navasco.

I found Navasco very refreshing and studied all subjects. It was also a school that was very much involved in soccer, field hockey, and drama; and I participated in both the drama club and the debating team even though I was a very shy young man.

Academic Achievement and an AFS International High School Exchange Student Scholarship Award in Navasco.

I began to academically shine in the school in my fourth year. I had gone to the school garden where I was very interested in agriculture. One of the students who had come to the garden indicated that my English teacher was looking for me. He did not, however, know why, and he had instructed students to find me. Suddenly I heard a motorcycle roaming toward the garden in the school. It was my English teacher who was a British expatriate. He indicated that he wanted me to participate in an essay competition being offered to all secondary schools in the country. "The reward of it is that if you are finally chosen among the eleven male and female students, then you will have an opportunity to go to the U.S. to study and complete your secondary school education, and you will also bring pride to our school, which desperately needs it", said Mr. E. Bresion. He handed me one of the applications and asked me why I did not enter the competition without him requesting I did. I told him that I had not heard of the competition. The class prefect who was in charge of informing the students about the essay competition had not yet done so. The English teacher wanted me to participate since l was one of the best English students not only in my class but all the three classes we had in form four. My heart began to palpitate. This was a young man who did not know people noticed, but here came the chief of the English department asking a young man to do something that prestigious, I mumbled to myself.

How could I refuse?

He offered me a ride back to the campus and told me he wanted to see the essay the next two days. I expressed my gratitude and went on to write the essay as a representative of Navasco. It was with pride and adulation that I was chosen, and I was not going to let this opportunity pass me by. I said to myself that with this opportunity I could also bring my school Navasco to the national picture if I won the essay competition. I completed the essay and handed my papers in.

In the same year the First Lady of the United States had visited Ghana, and the same English teacher requested three of his students to write a letter to Mrs. Nixon thanking her for coming to Ghana. I wrote a letter and never anticipated a reply but again was just happy that I was chosen. I completely forgot that I had written the letter. After about four months, my English teacher brought a letter to me from Mrs. Nixon as a reply to the letter I had written. He said, "Think about it. Thousands and thousands of people write to the First Lady of the USA every day, and she took the time to answer your letter." He assumed it was because I was clear with my ideas and she could read your penmanship. I was in cloud nine after I had the reply from Mrs. Nixon. Her letter was read to me by my English teacher who was more than flabbergasted about me getting a reply from the First Lady. He was very proud of his teaching.

I entered the competition and was one of eleven students chosen to represent Ghana after going through local-, district-, regional-, and national-level competition.

This competition was undertaken by the American Field Service organization, which had chapters throughout the world.

The competition also gave me the first-time opportunity to travel to the southern part of Ghana. It was there that I began to see the disparity between the southern and the northern parts of the Republic of Ghana. On the day of the national interview, Agambila and I were advised by the headmaster of Navasco to wear our school uniform, which consisted of a pair of khaki shorts and a white T-shirt with the

Navascan logo printed on the upper portion of the T-shirt. Whilst we were walking barefooted, there were other students who were being brought to the interview venue in all assortment of expensive cars, and the students came in all assortment of clothing I had never seen before. Agambila looked up to me as if to ask me what we were doing in the mix of this elegancy and show of wealth. I knew I was poor, and this was an opportune time to shine for my own pride and ego and a chance for the two of us to put Navasco on a national and international pedestal in Accra. Somehow I was not deterred. I told Agambila that we were going to beat all the rich students. I was used to these kinds of scenarios because I often got cookies and other assortment of snacks from well-to-do students in exchange for teaching or tutoring them. What I thought as rich in my part of the country was nothing compared to what I was seeing in Accra, the capital city of Ghana. The interview was held in the auspices of the Ministry of Education offices in Accra, the capital city of the Republic of Ghana. There were about six interviewers asking questions up and down the place, and I confidently answered all the questions to the best of my ability. I had expected to be very nervous in the midst of all strangers; but I was rather cool, calm, and confident.

After the interview, we went back to the International Student Hostel and prepared to go back to Navasco to await the final American Field Service International Essay Competition results.

All throughout this period including participating in the essay competition and all my travels for interview, I did not inform my siblings or parents. I did not want any encouragement or negativity during this critical stage of a national competition. I explained to my headmaster that I wanted to do this for myself. Navasco was at that time headed by Mr. McDonald who was a British expatriate who took us into his wing because he was proud that two of his Navascans were in a national competition who were about to attain national and international honors for the first time in the history of the school. This added to the reason I did not tell my parents because I did not have to ask for money for transportation because the headmaster and the school paid all our expenses.

The next day we left to go back to school early in the morning. It was announced on the national radio that eleven students were chosen, and as soon as we heard our names, we were overjoyed. Instead of rejoicing, I began to cry out of joy. I cannot up-to-date remember my trip back to school because I cried myself to sleep at the back of the school truck as we drove past the interior of Ghana.

We were welcomed back to school with pride and jubilation.

The night I arrived I sat down and wrote letters to my parents and sibling that I had obtained an American field Service Scholarship (AFS) to go to complete my high school education in the United States of America.

My father replied to my letter with the proudest letter he had ever written me, but my mother could not grasp the importance and enormity of this achievement and the distance of travel that was to follow.

School life was never the same. We were to go for medical examination and also to stay with host families in Ghana from the United States of America to familiarize ourselves with the American way of life before embarking on our trip to the country to finish the high school curriculum. At this stage I was in form four and had one more year in form five to complete my secondary school education in Ghana. This meant after one year in the United States of America, I had to come back to Ghana and complete my studies in form five before I could complete the secondary school program in Ghana. Essentially my classmates would be ahead of me when I came back. Was I ready for the sacrifice?

I went to Navrongo Hospital for my medical examination in preparation for my trip to the United States of America. After several weeks of taking the medical examination, I was called to report to the Navrongo General Hospital for the results. The medical officer and physician at that time was Dr. Kumar who was the father of a classmate and a friend of mine by the name of Nikhil Kumar. Dr. Kumar called me to his office and told me that my skin strip test was positive for a disease of the eyes called onchocerciasis or river blindness. Onchocerciasis is caused by a bite by the black fly and mosquitoes. It affects the optic nerves that can result in blindness. Dr. Kumar, even though he was Indian, said, "Son, I am very proud of your achievement and love you and respect you, but I am not going to rubber stamp your medical certificate that you have passed the medical exam when you have not. You maintaining your eyesight is more important to me than your travel to America where it is not a known disease entity," said Dr. Kumar.

I went blank and did not seem to understand what Dr. Kumar had said because of his accent and intonation. I politely asked him to repeat what he had just told me.

He again said that I did not pass the medical exam and for the first time added that it was going to affect my ability to take a trip to the United States of America.

By this time, it did not occur to me that Dr. Kumar was telling me that I could not go on my scholarship experience. He held my hand and said, "Son, you later in life will appreciate the decision we are making for you to get treatment rather than travel and not get the appropriate treatment abroad." He sat down and went through how to take the medication that was needed and their side effect.

At this time I was neither listening nor paying any attention to what Dr. Kumar was telling me.

"How can you do this to me?" I asked Dr. Kumar.

I exclaimed and suddenly became afraid and helpless.

I was done and did not have my beloved mother who had a magic way of making tragedies into something different.

I still had some courage to say thank you to Dr. Kumar, and with a heavy heart, I went back to my dormitory. I did not share the news with anybody because Dr. Kumar wanted me to keep it quiet in case he had a solution with the AFS International that could assure him that onchocerciasis would not affect my sight and compromise my lifelong plans.

We were left with about a week to go to the end of the school year. I immediately left school with the permission of my headmaster for my village Bulbia, where l always felt at home, the day we were dismissed for the summer holiday or long vacation as we knew it. As soon as I put my luggage from my head down, my mother started crying. I had not written home to tell my parents about my medical examination results, and I wondered how she knew what happened to me, I asked myself.

She told me that she had dreamt about my not being able to go on my scholarship because they did not have the money to pay my way to Accra and definitely to the United States of America. As if in trance, I held my mother and told my parent that I had won a full scholarship, which included food and clothing and they did not have to worry about not being able to afford to help me. I also then told them what Dr. Kumar told me my health not being in the best of shape, and he would not allow me to go to the United States because in America where they did not know what River blindness was, which could subsequently lead to my being blind.

"Isn't that your friend's father?" asked my mother.

"Are you sure he is not doing this because he does not want you to travel and wish it was his son?" said my mother. I could see she was not pleased. After I answered her questions to her satisfaction, I expected my mother to start insulting Dr. Kumar. Instead she held my hand and sat me down on her lap; by then she was sitting on the floor as if I was still the crippled child she had raised. She said that she was thankful to Allah and our ancestors for helping Dr. Kumar to diagnose me in the early stages of the disease.

She had experience with oncho because a lot of young and able boys and girls were already blind from the disease in my village Bulbia. She prayed with me and asked my younger sister to get me some water to drink since I had just walked from a twelve-mile journey. My mother also indicated that my ancestors probably were not pleased. I was going away to a fresh land, so she would discuss it with my uncles to pray and pour libation for me to our ancestors. I stayed the whole summer vacation in my village Bulbia and went farming and looking for medicinal herbs and roots with my uncles. At the end of the summer vacation, I went back to Walewale, the nearest town, to go back to school.

In Walewale I was inundated with questions as to why I was not in America already.

I did not know that this achievement was considered to be a whole tribal affair or business. Many people encouraged me to get healthy, and everybody I met assured me that I would win subsequent scholarships as if they were the overseers of the AFS International Organization. A lot of people came with well-wishes and indicated that they were praying for me to get healthy.

I arrived in school in August 1970 with some students delighted that I was back in school while others were very sarcastic about it. Finally about a week in school in the assembly hall the headmaster explained to the entire student body why I was not already in the United States. The headmaster went ahead and assured the students that he had no doubt that I would be going in 1971. I wondered who assured my headmaster of this confidence. Then he said something that I never thought before that I felt that it was a blessing because I would have an opportunity to complete my education at the ordinary level (G.C.E. 'O' level) examination, which heralds the end of secondary school education next year before going to the United States.

He was very confident I would be chosen since he said my essay and interview still was one of the best selected.

If my headmaster wanted to get a monster off my back and head, he did, and the burden of having to explain to each and every individual was taken off my head also. I came in tune with my situation and started school again. I concentrated on my studies. I was also at this time very religious and spent a lot of time praying, be it in Islam, Christianity or praying to my ancestors through deities contrary to my modern upbringing. I became a Roman Catholic and was baptized into the Catholic faith. I was in charge of all religious activities within Navasco. At one time I had contemplated on becoming a priest until I went to America and saw some of the hypocrisies of modern religion.

I studied hard for the O-level examination even amidst a student strike that we had in Navasco. I for once could not see why students were striking because of food the Ghana government could not supply when these students and their own parents could not feed the striking students at home.

It was amazing to see how healthy students were when they were in the school for three months. When the same students went home to their villages, they often came back skinny and malnourished due to lack of proper nutrition, yet the same students organized a strike because the school could not supply the students with plantain.

The slogan of the strike was "We don't want kenkey, Macdonald kenkey," since the school constantly supplied the students with kenkey (made from corn). Most of the strike leaders were back at the GCE (advance level) A level and did not have much to do in school. I felt I had a lot to do to come to par with the ring leaders, and I was not ready to forfeit that opportunity. I did not see a need to follow the masses, and I left the school. When the school was eventually closed due to the food strike, I went back to my village to study for my final external examination. Since my village was without electricity, I studied mainly during the daylight. I had no electricity to study. At times I used candles, but I was limited as to the length of time the candlestick could last, and also the smoke from the candles always caused my eyes to burn. On one occasion I fell asleep and almost got myself engulfed in smoke when the lit candle fell on my bed sheet.

My last year in Navrongo Secondary School was one of my best years in my life. I was very quiet, religious, and reserved. I concentrated on my studies. This year I was also a lot healthier, and my risk of losing my eyesight was very much minimized because I had undergone oral therapy for onchocerchiasis, which was by itself brutal in terms of their side effects.

It was also this year that I re-entered the AFS scholarship program, and again I won the competition in 1971. I was one of the eleven students who proudly represented my country, Ghana, in an educational and social student exchange program.

I was informed by the AFS International representative that I was to stay with a family in Bloomer, Wisconsin. I did not know much about the state of Wisconsin or the small town of Bloomer.

My research in the school library and the Bolgatanga Regional library, which had just opened, did not yield any information about the city of Bloomer, but I knew about the geography and landscape of the state of Wisconsin. After not finding much on Bloomer, Wisconsin, I almost concluded that I was being sent from Bulbia, Ghana, to a similar village in the United States of America.

It was ironical that my family consisted of almost all females and that I was to be a host student to a family with all girls.

This year it was assumed that I was going to make the trip to the United States of America, but I knew I wanted to get back to complete my secondary school education and get into the advance level of Ghana's secondary school systems and subsequently to attain entry into a university.

About three weeks prior to leaving to the United States, I left Bulbia to stay with an American host family in Accra, All the students and most of the host families in Accra were made to tour Cape Coast; the Akosombo Dam (the second largest man-made dam in the world); and some of the numerous castles in Cape Coast, Elmina, and Takoradi. These castles reminded me of the vestiges of slavery; and I was very uncomfortable about them because most of my tribesmen were captured, sold, and became slaves to endure inhumane treatment on a trip I was going without any beating, chains, or humiliation. The visit to the castles was a very, very bitter experience; but the trip molded me to be tolerant, respectful, and forgiving to slave masters and tribes that participated in enslaving people.

I asked myself questions such as why was this form of brutality allowed to even happen?

Who was to be blamed, and how cruel were human beings to one another?

At the dungeons and at "the point of no return" where President Obama went when he was in Ghana, it was so dark that it seemed as if it was the end of the world. The irony to slavery was that beside the area of no return, there was a church. I wondered what the slave masters were praying for. Definitely it was not for the well-being of the slaves who were bound like packs of sardine. I often heard my father talking about slavery and the role our villages played, but it was never a kid's conversations; and even though I was curious, I was often shut down with my father's famous statement, "You are too young for the elderly person's conservation." I wanted to know more, but my father sometimes looked to me that the topic of slavery, which our tribe was part of, brought pain and sorrow in his eyes. I felt my father was hiding something and was very uncomfortable about it. I once asked him why the history of slavery was not being taught in school at the primary, middle, and secondary school levels. He never replied to me till he died in 1994. After going to these castles, I started being homesick even though I had been going to boarding schools all my life. I could hear my mother's words to me when she dropped me at the lorry station to take a bus, "Do not fight or argue with those people because I hear they love the gun. If somebody hurts you or wants to argue, move away from the person and pray for the person." At the lorry station, she also told me not to forget the promise I made to her about my older brother's drinking problem, She grabbed me, looked at me at an angle, and said to me, "I know you will be good to me, your father, your grandmother, your village, tribe, and the whole of Ghana."

My mother looked into my eyes and reiterated, "Don't forget that a coward always lives to tell a story the next day, but a brave man is often mourned and honored with parades and medals, which he will never enjoy. The nice words said after a brave man's funeral cannot replace the loss of a grieving mother and father." I nodded my head and promised my mother that what she had taught me was not going to be left in vain.

I suddenly remembered my crippled and disabled days and saw the strong-witted and never-yielding mother who brought me along in life. It is not customary for a son to hug his mother in my culture, but I could not help it. My mother had gone through a lot with me, and I love her so much. As if the wind blew me to my mother, I gave her a hug, and both of us started crying in unison.

The bus gradually pulled out of the lorry station, and something said to me, "Son you are all alone; and I will watch to see if you keep everything your father and mother, siblings, and the entire Kantonsi and Mamprugu had taught you." I nodded, and proudly the tears drained, and the sense of pride came upon me.

After our visits to the castles and some zoos in Kumasi, we returned to our host families in preparation to take our trip to the United States.

This was considered an orientation program. We learnt about the different foods, customs, and high school life in the United States by watching movies.

At the last night before we left, we had a meeting in preparation to leave.

Life in America an an AFS International High School Exchange Student and the testing of my Catholic Faith and believes.

O n or about the 27th of August 1971 bright and early in the morning, I woke up in a luxurious home I was not used to. I was used to lying on the floor with my *zana* mat and cloth.

One would think that I would ache less on the bed and be much more comfortable, but I tossed all night and woke up more tired than the day before. All the students gathered at the AFS coordinator's home, and we were driven to the airport. My mind started wondering all over the place. This was to me my first and longest flight and the first time to leave the state of Ghana.

Every preparation for the flight was handled by the coordinators of the AFS International, and I had not much to carry aboard. When I got inside the plane, it was huge; but when I saw all the students of my age, I all of a sudden became relieved. In the plane the first student I met was from South Africa followed by a Libyan student. I was told by the white South African student that if we were to go to South Africa, we the Black African students would not be allowed out of the airplane due to his country's policy of apartheid. As a student of Marcus Garvey, Kwame Nkrumah, and L'Ouverture, he did not have to give me any explanation. I was a student and strong believer in Pan-Africanism and considered all Africans as brothers and sisters. I insisted that he told me more about South Africa and its people even though he was white and belonged to the subjugating class. He was apologetic for some of the policies of his country's system of minority rule. I looked at him, and we continued our conversation as to the future of our beloved continent.

We jumped up and down the plane as if we were on the earth. There was no thought of danger in my mind, and no other students showed any grave concerns. The busier I kept myself, the more I was not tempted to think of my mother and siblings I was leaving behind in Ghana. I was determined not to get homesick.

We arrived into New York City, and we were met by other AFS International officers. We were directed into buses at the John F. Kennedy Airport in New York City and taken to C. W. Post College in Long Island, New York. Here we again met even more students from all over the world. It was a beautiful and colorful event as the students with all shades of color made the world smaller as a gentle breeze blew across the school's parking lot.

We barely got any sleep, but we really didn't care. We went into orientation before leaving New York City for our host towns. Three days later, I was on a Greyhound bus on my way to Bloomer, Wisconsin, which I later found out was known as the "rope jump" capital of the world.

I kept trying to imagine how big Bloomer was when I could not find it on the world map on several occasions I had viewed during my research.

On arrival in Eau Claire, Wisconsin, at the Greyhound bus station, we were again met by local AFS International organizers and my host family and other host families; and there began my American experience, which will eternally define my life.

From Eau Claire to Bloomer, which is a twelve-mile journey, I could not keep my eyes open because I was exhausted from all the good times I had with all the other students. We arrived at 1638 Riggs Street, in a green corner house where my American host family resided.

I was taken to my room and introduced to my two American sisters who had come with their families to meet me. My first two American sisters were already married, and one was a student at

University of Wisconsin—Eau Claire in the city of Eau Claire, Wisconsin. This began the second chapter of my life, and I was excited by the way it started.

After a short conversation with my host parents, I went to bed and woke up early in the morning in a brand-new environment. It was summertime or nearly the fall, but to me it was as if I had just flown into the thickness and darkness of winter. My American mother who became like my own mother, sensing that I was cold, got me a jacket. I was not shy to wear a jacket at the tail end of the summer period because I was genuinely cold. Whenever I walked along Ridge Street from east to west, I often saw children either drawing their parents' attention or pointing fingers at me. I began to draw parallels to when I was a baby and saw a white man (Dr. Faile of Nalerigu Baptist Medical Center) for the first time in my life. We the kids would often scream and run and call the name 'Broni' whilst looking for shelter. When I saw the same thing happening to me in Bloomer and how I felt with people calling me names and running, I genuinely felt bad and ashamed for seeing similar things being done in my environs to people who looked different. As a kid in Ghana, there was no racial intent behind what the kids did. As a crippled child, I had gone through all forms of abuse and did not want to see it especially when my mother was not around to give me a pep talk. Some of the kids were genuinely mean, calling me nigger, and started running. Unknown to me at this juncture was that there were no black families in Bloomer, Wisconsin. Several calls were placed to my host house when they saw me going in there to enquire as to my presence. Initially, full members of the AFS International club knew of my arrival, but I later found out that a lot of people were very curious because they thought a black family had moved into the city of Bloomer. Calls were even made to several places within the city of Bloomer environs to enquire about my presence in the town. My American mother, Mrs. Victor Olson, who is a sensitive woman but very astute, decided to publicize my presence using the local media that a foreign exchange student was going to spend a year in Bloomer High School. The news bulletin included my background, my family background, and my future aspirations. When I arrived, my American parents were Methodists, and I was a mass-serving Catholic. I often accompanied my American family to their church activities.

The Methodist Church of Bloomer, which I did not actually belong to, and its pastor accommodated me more and contributed in making my one-year stay in Bloomer more pleasant. My attitude toward Christianity was to take a drastic change in this small town. As aforementioned, I grew up in a family where my mother has always been a Moslem and my parents did not push religion into our throats. l was very close to my mother because we had gone through a lot together. She agreed for me to concentrate on going to the English or Western-style schools since it did not seem I was involved too deeply in Islamic preaching and duties. I therefore went on and involved myself in the Catholic Church. I was very impressed with the patience and exemplary life of Father John from Bolgatanga. I also felt at peace whenever I went to church, and I could understand God's teaching and the Bible's impact on the social life of humans and life after death. This is the background of my conversion into Catholicism. My father did not object to my decision so far as I participated in pouring libation and respected his paganism. Most people who often became educated would often convert to Christianity either through their own will or through pressure exerted on them by Christian missionaries. My father, even though he was one of the well educated few, was too ethnocentric to convert. He believed in his paganism/animism till he died in nineteen-ninety six. When I got to Bloomer, Wisconsin I was more than willing to continue my religious endeavors. I strongly believed that somebody higher up had guided my life up to this point. I also strongly believed that Jesus was part of my adolescence. I often would alternate the Methodist Church with the Catholic Church that I thought I belonged. On one Sunday after attending church and serving mass, a priest whom l do not wish to remember his name, walked up to me and started to carry out a conversation with me. He explained to me that the Bloomer Catholic Church was beginning to lose its congregation, and I asked him if I had anything to do with the drop in his congregation's numbers. He told me how he was really impressed with my enthusiasm and my desire to participate in church activities as a true Christian is expected, but he then added that he had been getting complaints from his congregation about me being a mass server as a black man. I pretended that I did not hear what he had just told me. The statement came to my chest like a bolt of lightning or thunder. I had expected entities relative to race relations because I had read about great people like Booker T. Washington, Stokely Carmichael (whom I later treated as a patient in the island of Grenada), and Ms. Angela Davis whom I admired and adored as a kid and still adores her up-to-date. In several aspects my own mother, who was uneducated from the Western point of view and did not even know which part of the world I was going, warned me about race relations. Even though I was not surprised that a black mass server was not welcomed by Catholic priest, it still came to me as a shock because it was coming from a representative of God on earth. Was I surprised? No, a flash of light came over me and reminded me that in the horrors of slavery, there was a church at the 'point of no return' in the slave castle where human beings were savagely beaten, chained, and starved but yet were expected to survive on the long journey across the Atlantic Ocean to America. This priest apparently declared me persona non grata in the same church he had prayed to God for forgiveness. I equated his nonacceptance to the same savagery that my ancestors had gone through solely because we were born black by the same God that he claimed to be a representative of. Somehow the priest expected me to be angry; but I took a deep breath, looked around as if my mother was present, and without uttering a word I walked proudly and meticulously out of the mass server's dressing room and went into the congregation. As I sat down, I looked around the church and said to myself, "Are these the same people who are complaining about a young Negro serving mass in a Catholic Church in which some of the first popes of the Church were Negroid like me? I said to myself that probably this Congregation did not know about Pope Gelasius I, the forty-ninth Pope, Pope Victor II, the twelfth Pope and Pope Miltrades the thirty-second Pope and all the Carthaginians who martyred and were the backbone of the Catholic Church. In my mind this was the thought of one person supposedly serving the Lord. Why should I succumb to somebody who wanted to react unpleasantly to a decision he thought was the right thing to do for his church and his congregation? Probably I thought it was an economic one because the few people that showed up in church, the less monetary collections will be made by the priest; and on top of that, I had no donations to give to the church. The smaller the number of people showing up in church because of the presence of one unfortunate Black boy, the less the donations and the smaller the church's coffers. I tried to make excuses for the priest. The more I thought about it, the more the point of no return in the Cape Coast Castle kept coming back to remind me how wicked we humans can be to each other. Somehow, the small churches that were next to the point of no return (when slaves could not return) were also symbols that represented God's hatred to mankind, but they were used as a façade for the slaves to think that God was watching them even in time of hopelessness. After the service, I walked home, and throughout my journey to Riggs Street, I kept praying about what to tell my host mother. I had learnt in such a short period how my host mother would react, so I decided to keep things to myself. I would only bring something up if I had no solution to the problem or if I felt it would not cause friction between my host parents and the Bloomer populace since I had to live in this community for only one year and my host family had to still live in the community after I left.

On this day, i felt the world was falling apart because on my way home after being told a Negro could not serve mass as a mass server, as I was on my way home as I crossed the main street from a new fast food stand that had just opened across the Bloomer High School., I turned on a corner and after a short walk from the main bridge in downtown Bloomer an old lady was trying to cross the street. She was slow and seemed to have stopped in the middle of the road, I saw vehicles ploughing toward the old lady. I walked toward her to give her a helping hand across the street because I was afraid she was going to be ploughed down by the oncoming cars. As I came toward her, I realized that a vehicle was coming toward us, and she had a hard time crossing the street. I helped her cross the street, and she raised her head up as if to see who was helping her. She said no word of thanks to me. She, however, had a stern and scornful look and gave me a short unfriendly smile and then looked back down. After knowing she had successfully crossed the street and was out of danger, I started to walk. She called out to me. "Boy, come here. I want to ask you a question," exclaimed the old lady. I slowed down and walked back to her. She looked at me and told me that her Jesus was a white one and not a black Jesus. In order to understand what she was saying since she was also walking at a very slow pace, I slowed down to listen to her. As I came close to her, I stopped in respect as is done in my culture to the elderly. She walked toward me and asked me which part of the town my family lived, and she wanted to know what I was doing in Bloomer. In not hesitating and not giving me time to answer her question, she told me to go to where my fellow colored people were living. I was waiting for an opportune time to answer, but before I could open my mouth, she asked if I worshipped the same God she did. As quickly as I heard the words and knowing where the conversation was heading to, I could hear my mother in Africa advising me not to disrespect or respond to her. I looked at her and said a prayer for this frail elderly female who just wanted somebody to pour her frustrations on. Whilst I was praying, she asked me what l was doing. I told her that I was praying and that even though I was black, l was being protected by the God who foresaw her too. She told me I was wrong. I did not, however, want to prolong this conversation since l wholeheartedly felt I was eventually going to say something unpleasant to this frail lady contrary to what my mother had taught me.

I told her that I had been sent on an errand by my American mother and emphasized that it was imperative that I got home promptly. As I started to move, she looked startled; and after about a hundred feet away from her, I looked back at her, and she did not seem to have any desire to move. I even wondered if she could walk.

I went home undressed, but the episode remained in my mind to tell my host mother about it because I suspected she would find who it was and confront them. I did not want my American mother to be burdened with these problems, and secondarily I did not feel she had a solution to it. I, however, was a lot closer to my American mother than my host daddy as it was in my own household.

The rest of the day was a long day. In the evening I then decided to walk toward Chippewa Falls, which had a lot fewer people, and I had more free time to pray and reflect on the day's events. When I came back from walking, I saw my American dad watching a game. It was a preseason game in American football. I sat with him and watched the game and he did well explaining to me the rules of the game. Even with his explanation of the rules of the game, I had a hard time understanding the rules and necessary regulations that were involved. We spoke about soccer and how it was popular in my secondary School in Ghana and the world at large except in the United States of America.

He explained some rules of the game to me and indicated that there was a position on the football team that Bloomer High School could use me as a student place kicker if I was interested. I continued to watch football every Sunday and Monday nights and gradually fell in love with the game. The Monday after I had discussed with my host dad about my interest in the game, I walked past the school field where the students were practicing late in the evening, and the game fascinated me. I soon became interested in playing, but quickly it hit me like lightning the fact that I did not walk for a lot of my life, and I was trying to get myself in what I thought was a brutal game. I did not participate in sporting activities in Ghana mainly because of fear of injuring myself in the legs.

I also thought that by taking up a sport it could help me mentally and physically in order to make the year a fruitful one.

I also wanted to use this year to participate in activities be it sports or school subjects that I did not have the opportunity in my secondary school in Ghana. After visiting the football session and not understanding it, I went back home in near darkness; and after discussing with my American father, I decided to participate in some sporting activity. This to me was an interesting turnaround in my life because whilst in secondary school in Ghana I hardly took part in sporting activities mainly because when you were not a superb athlete, other students often mocked students with less athletic ability.

I was known and nicknamed Socrates or an academician but not as a sports person. I often ran cross-country or long-distance running only to find myself in the back of the pack. So my decision to participate in sporting activities caught me by surprise. The following day I went to the football coach to inform him I was interested in playing American football.

AFS International also had their own rules about involvement of students in contact sports. The kicker position was a safe position, and I was not permitted to punt or return kicks because of concerns that I would get hurt.

The day school started, my American family with my American sister, Betty, went to school with me. My host house was within walking distance even though it seemed so far walking in the snow. In school I was a subject of curiosity and intrigue.

I wore my spectacles, and now according to my children, I looked like Steve Urkel then.

I had numerous questions as to where I came from.

When did you leave Africa?

Where did your family live, and how big is your tree?

What kind of food do you eat in Africa?

How did you get to America? asked another student.

I would look and look with amazement as to the type of questions that were being asked.

Initially I thought these questions were either too childish or full of ignorance. Some of the questions about Tarzan and primitive life really tested my patience. After two weeks of starting classes, it gradually occurred to me that the questions were appropriate for the amount of knowledge on Africa. I initially thought that it was solely done for me to test my patience and/or knowledge, but as I got into the high school within two weeks, I figured that most Americans did not know much of world history or geography.

I was amazed how little American students knew about Africa and how Africans lived was equaled to life in Tarzan movies that were made right here in the United States of America and were very popular in the country in the early 1970s. l went to school and registered and took subjects I did not know much about. I also took advantage of the time I had by joining the debating and forensic teams.

I ended up writing research papers and presented my essays at the district and state forensic championship that took place in the capital city of Madison, Wisconsin. I also made the honor roll in my school. Some of the students could not understand how an African could surpass their capabilities because they had preconceived and inbred thoughts that blacks we not intelligent human beings but were very good in sports. I enjoyed my forensic club membership, and as a member of the Future Farmers of America Club, since Bloomer is predominantly a farming community, I learnt a lot not about farming alone but also about agro–business.

In the fall I participated as a place kicker in the school varsity football team. During practice I was not allowed contact sport because I had to be protected as an exchange student. The AFS International Organization was very protective of the exchange students because of the risk of injuries, but also I later found that it was very costly to the AFS International when an exchange student got hurt. I had joined the team as a place kicker and punter, but the punter position was taken away from me because of the above concerns. The kicker was given to me because it did not involve contact sports, I thought. I was later to find out what a mistake that was during a game when I was tackled down rather violently by a two-hundred-and-seventy-five-pound linebacker from Chetek. I took such a vicious hit, but when I got up, I started laughing; but definitely I was still in pain and felt it. After giving me a vicious hit, he said, "Welcome to American football," and added that this was not soccer. I braved it after the hit, got up, made a facial gesture to the Chetek player, and then rejoined the huddle .

We lost most of our games in 1971, but I was perfect in all my extra points and field goal kicks. The most interesting thing was when I kicked one extra point to win our homecoming game. The whole town became lively with parades, and a lot of people from Bloomer enjoyed the win and the celebration that followed.

Then came the prom, which my American mother insisted I needed to go with a "date." It was quite an experience, and it was to be the first time I went out with a girl all alone and not being escorted by my junior brother who was always coaxed by my sisters to come with me.

In school there was tremendous amount of pressure on me to drink alcohol or drugs. Even in the 1970s in small-town Bloomer these vices were available. Several attempts and pressure were placed on me just to try, but I was very insistent on my refusal not to break a promise I had made to my mother, God, ancestors and myself. On one occasion after a football game the whole team, cheerleaders and ancillary staff went hay riding; there was so much pressure put on me that in order to fit the norm I washed a can of Miller beer with water and filled it with soda and started to drink. Some of the kids, thinking I was drinking beer started to cheer me on. I often asked myself why fellow students were so bent on seeing me drink alcohol when it was so clear that I was taught by my parents not to. The more I was pushed to smoke marijuana and drink beer, the more convinced that I was doing the right thing. "Your mother is not here to see you drink. Why don't you just take a sip?" said Rob. I looked around and could feel my mother's presence. When they could not get me to do what they wanted me to do, some of the students never invited me again, or I made up my mind not to go to places where I did not fit the alcohol or smoking model. I often got away by emptying empty cans of beer and filling them with water and pretended to be drinking alcohol with my friends to let them feel I was part of the group enjoyed my water and as a consequence never got into any problems surrounding the use of alcohol or drugs. There was tremendous pressure from fellow football players and other students inducing me to smoke illicit drugs and drink alcohol since I had never done it before.

There was one occasion after a football game when we had gone hay riding and everybody got drunk except me. However, when the police came up, they started questioning me expecting me to be drunk. I told the officer to taste beer from my can. When he found out that it was water and that I did not smell of alcohol, he let me go.

In my mind my mother's words were always my protection. My mother made me promise that I was not going to go into drinking alcohol or smoking as my senior brother did. She often spoke about the evils of smoking and the effect of all the smoke and fumes on the body. She advised me the effect peer pressure could have in getting one to do things they did not intend to do. As a young boy, I was often reminded of the pain and agony and humiliation my parents especially my mother went through because my senior brother drank and smoked which eventually destroyed his life. Alcohol consumption caused chronic pancreatitis and eventually killed my handsome and intelligent senior brother. Any discussions or reading about alcohol often brings back memories of my brother. On one occasion, when my senior brother was a teacher in Doba Middle school, located in a small town in the now Upper West Region of Ghana, I visited him during one of my school holidays. My brother often took me to help him in teaching and grading his students' lessons and tests, and he also was very proud of my academic achievements and did not hesitate to boast about it. On one occasion, he sent me to go and buy him a packet of cigarettes, which I did; but when I returned to his apartment (room with veranda), he was not home. I saw an old stump of cigarettes on the floor that was left burning on the veranda floor. I quickly picked up the small piece and began to inhale. Suddenly I got a very nasty slap from behind me.

My bother hit the small pieces of cigarette from my hand and almost broke my hand. After hitting the cigarette off by mouth, my bother said, "I do not want our mother to blame me for influencing you to start smoking cigarettes. I have disappointed our parents enough." He did not want me to go through the path he went through.

Since then I made a promise whilst crying to him that I would never drink alcohol or smoke cigarettes and all the things that go along. I respected my brother very much for not wanting me to emulate him since he knew it was wrong, yet he had no willpower to stop being influenced by his peers.

I made a lot of friends playing American football and also did a lot of traveling during football season to towns and villages such Chetek, Hayward, and numerous others in the state of Wisconsin.

I also participated in short- and long-distance running, but I did not enjoy it as much as I did American football. Sports played an important role in my life as an exchange student and was instrumental in making my stay in Bloomer, Wisconsin, very worthwhile. I made up my mind to participate in events and took classes I did not have the opportunity to participate in my country and at the same time enjoy myself rather than be homesick.

When I arrived in Bloomer High School, I participated in Forensics and debating. I took part in the district and state forensic championship in the Madison, Wisconsin, where I presented a document on the *Pentagon Papers*. I was fascinated of the Nixon family because Mrs. Nixon responded to my letter after her visit to Ghana in 1970.

Even though I never personally met Mr. Nixon, after writing and presenting a paper on the *Pentagon Papers*, I often wondered in my mind what would happen if the anonymous person involved in writing the story had some personal vendetta against the Nixons and just wanted to destroy them.

In school I enjoyed myself and studied subjects I had no prior knowledge.

I also missed my family in Ghana and had a lot of difficulty with the food and water. In the first few weeks after I got into the United States, I ended up in a Bloomer hospital. I was hospitalized after I developed severe diarrhea and became very dehydrated, and this was attributed to the change in food and water. Being used to eating everything cooked fresh and nothing refrigerated and not used to eating cold foods, I found my stomach hurting and cramping whenever I ate. On one occasion, whilst we were eating, I was having a lot of abdominal cramps and pains; my American mother looked up to me and asked me how I liked the food in America. Without thinking and without hesitation, I told her how horrible the food was because my stomach was hurting.

I regretted later on saying that because my American mother took it that I did not like her cooking, which was absolutely not true. I had not yet learnt the political aspects of speaking in America and found out that the free colloquial expressions I used at home in Ghana where one did not have to be political did not apply. My American mother did not seem to forget my ill-concerned answer, and I learnt very quickly not to be so blunt in my expressions. After hospitalization in Bloomer General Hospital, I got better and gradually became used to the food and hence enjoyed the food. I also began to think of medicine as a goal after my hospitalization because the doctor was kind and very professional. "What do you want to be in the future?" asked the doctor. I immediately said to him that I wanted to be a doctor just like him. He smiled, shook my hand, and walked away.

In Bloomer most of the students who were involved with the student exchange activities in general were girls and most of the boys did not actively involve themselves. I also found out that the girls were more outgoing and anxious and wanting to learn about other cultures than the boys. In school activities involving dancing, one would always find the boys sitting together and the girls in the middle of the dance hall dancing by themselves. It was very fascinating to find that this was very different from my secondary school in Ghana.

In secondary school in Ghana, it was always the most popular, athletic, or rich students who dressed well and could get dates with our very few girls who were often in the middle of the dance hall enjoying themselves and participating in the dancing activities.

At this stage in my life, I was considered a bookworm, and no girls would ever look at bookworms who didn't have an athletic build. At one time I got upset about being called names that I would discuss things with my stepmother Adisa who always told me, "Son, go and study. The same girls who don't want you today will surely want you in the future when you are successful in life." I would smile and go about my work.

My shyness gradually dissipated as I had to deal with an organization that was predominantly female. Most of my best friends were female, and my two best friends I have had to date in school were Debbie Feiten and Bonnie Doyle. Bonnie and Debbie were both my neighbors, and they became my two best friends. My stay in Bloomer would not have been as good without Bonnie's intuition, advice, and help.

She had a purple Pinto car, and since she was a year older, she could drive. She showed me around places such as Chippewa Falls and other surrounding small towns and farmlands I could not have had the opportunity to know. Her mother and father were also great people, and I understood that curiously because Bonnie's brother had just returned from the Vietnam War and was having a lot of adjustment problems, which I could relate to and which her family understood very much. I became very close to Mrs. Doyle. Words cannot express the gratitude I owe to these great friends of mine. There were things I could share with them that I could not share with my American mother and father. My youngest host sister, Betty, was a freshman; and as such, we did not have much in common.

On weekends we had gatherings in different towns involving the AFS International exchange students. During these meetings, we learnt a lot about ourselves and got to know more about the countries that were represented by the students. We played games, mainly soccer and ping-pong (table tennis), and we also had parties where we danced. Exchange students represented Greece, Tunisia, Colombia, West Germany, South Africa, and Ethiopia.

A lot of us missed home, but during the times we got together, one could not deduce that we were homesick from the friendships that we made.

These occasions were like a miniature United Nations, and we did have discussions as to how we could one by one or collectively work forward changing the world. The issues we discussed about was the role apartheid played in the liberation of South Africans at that time. Included in our group were white students from South Africa who educated us on some of the activities that were going on in South Africa.

Exchanging ideas and understanding each other were some of these items the AFS International exchange program taught us, and I was very grateful to have had the experience even though I came from a poor and meek environment.

What was amazing is that I thought that everybody came from the same poor background as I did. I found out that some of the students came from very wealthy homes and were used to having maids in their homes. The more I got to see the disparities in our lives, the more I became ever more grateful to my poor parents who brought us up to respect people and be humble. My mother often said that no matter who we were, we were all God's children.

My stay in Bloomer, Wisconsin, was essentially smooth except for the few items that I had earlier alluded to. Another person who made my stay worthwhile was my adopted aunt Ms. Elizabeth Nimtz who often came to my host family's house and often invited me to her house to converse. I became very close to her because I had discussion with her about things that were happening to me in Bloomer that I could not discuss with my host mother. I am forever grateful to her, and may she rest in peace.

Return to Ghana and G.C.E.
'A' Education in Navasco.

The year 1971 was a very busy year and passed by very quickly, and in several ways I grew and learnt a lot from this experience.

Some changes were welcomed, but others were often frowned upon. My attitude toward religion was one that had changed drastically. In my mind I know it was not God who had made me persona non grata in the Catholic Church. It was, however, hard to forget the frailties of humans even if those persons were the priests or clergy and were suppose to spread the goodwill of God to sinful man. I also reasoned that priest would rather sacrifice me rather than loose his congregation, which made up his economic base. I was young, and I rebelled by not going back to the Catholic Church in Bloomer, Wisconsin, but went to the Methodist Church with my American family. I reasoned that if the priest who stopped me from serving mass was a God-fearing person, it would not have been difficult for him to realize that he had hurt a child of God, and a gesture of finding out what had happened to me would have shown that he was really a representative of the Lord on earth. Could people who are stewards of religion be so far withdrawn from the teachings of God as to hurt the feelings of a young person? After thinking about it, I remembered what I had seen at the castles in Cape Coast, Ghana. Just above the 'point of no return' when chained and sometimes beaten and bleeding slaves had no choice but to go into slave ships but could not be returned to land no matter their mental or physical condition was a place of prayer. This is the epitome of religious mockery. I also said to myself, where is the church in South Africa? So I went back to Ghana without the same enthusiasm about religion as I had before I went to the United States of America.

The biggest change in me was that I was no longer shy in speaking to friends of the opposite sex since I had developed such good friends of the opposite sex in Bloomer.

Overall, my stay in Bloomer was one of the best experiences in my life, and it helped in making me what I am today.

My American mother, Ms. Victor Olson, helped me a lot. On one occasion my American family took me to an opera in Eau Claire even though I did not want to go. My American mother stood her ground, and I eventually went. I tried to rebel, but my American mother insisted. "I am your American mother, and you better do what I ask you to do," said my American mother. "You are part of this family, and you will participate in everything that we do," she added. The operas were very boring to me, but I could not express it. I, however, enjoyed the cultural experience, and never did I refuse to participate in any activity the family partook. My American mother was just as stern as my own mother, and I appreciated her and the entire Olson family.

My American mother was also instrumental in teaching me how to put on a tie for my senior prom amidst open opposition from me. Today, anytime I put on a tie, it often comes back to remind me the tantrum I threw when my American mother suggested that I learn how to put one on in conjunction with a suit. To me the ultimate symbol of Westernization was the tie, which I was not completely going to delve myself into. I am so glad and thankful that she insisted. "I will teach you how to dress up with a tie no matter what symbol it represented or did not represent to you," said my American mother. "Raising a child is not a democracy, and I call the shots, and all you can do is to listen to me, son," she added.

In late May 1971, my days to return to Ghana was fast approaching. I began to dream more about home. In the 1970s I could not readily call home because there were no phones in my village

Bulbia as they are now available everywhere today. My father often wrote me a couple of letters to keep me abreast with things at home. I also started thinking more about how to readjust to conditions in my country when I got back home to Ghana.

When the bus rolled in to pick us up, present were my host parents, my two American sisters Betty and Janice, and my two best friends Bonnie Doyle and Debbie Feiten. It was at this juncture that I showed some emotions by crying. It was mixed emotions because I was also very happy that I was going back to see my parents and siblings whom I really missed, but on the other hand, I was leaving my American mother and my best friends behind. It was the longest time I had ever been away from my loved ones.

I thanked and hugged my American parents and my friends and took my seat in the back of the bus so that everybody could see me wave goodbye when the bus started moving. I waved and waved until we were out of sight. At this time my mind was already focused on as to how fast I was going to get to Ghana, my dear homeland.

In late June 1972 i returned to Ghana in a very dignified position. Only my sister Sala, who was at this time a state-registered nurse, came to meet me at the Kotoka International Airport in Accra.

"Hello, Zara's crippled son," she joked. I walked proudly to her as if I had not heard her and gave my sister a hug. As I disembarked from the plane, I felt a sigh of relief that I had achieved something and that I was able to stay away from my family this long without involving myself in any problems that could not be managed unlike some of my fellow AFS international Exchange students who were sent back to their countries after they got into one trouble or the other.

I came back to Ghana knowing very well that I had passed my GCE O levels (general certificate of education ordinary level) examination with flying colors. The results were mailed to me by September 1971 by my younger brother after they were released by Navrongo Secondary School. I had one of the best grades in the school and the country and had attained a scholarship to attend my former school or my second and third choices of secondary schools that I could attend if I wanted to for the GCE A levels (general certificate of education advanced level) course. I came home from the United States knowing that I had to continue my secondary school education. I also had an American high school diploma from Bloomer High School.

I still had about six weeks to spend on holidays before returning to school. I stayed with my younger brother who had completed his secondary school education in Bawku Secondary School, a town now in the Upper East Region of the Country. He had started to work with Ghana Airways in Tamale, the capital city of the now Northern Region of Ghana.

I left for my village via Walewale. When I arrived in Walewale, I was treated as if I was somebody special, but I did not deem it so.

The whole Mamprugu and Kantonsi tribes were very proud that their son had represented the whole country with honor and dignity. Most people came to me when I was in the lorry station and welcomed me home as if I were a hero.

My mother somehow knew I had arrived in Walewale even though I did not want it broadcasted till I got home in order to surprise my mother. Even though there were no land or cell phones then, news at the local level traveled faster than one expected. The chief's talking drums were used to announce my arrival in Wungu, the traditional capital of the West Mamprusi District.

When I got to my village by lorry, my mother came just outside the village of Bulbia and brought with her all her magical incantations and brew in order to protect me. She always had a routine to welcome us home whenever we were back in the village. She believed that we had to be protected by our ancestors and Allah. She often prayed and poured libation to our deities for our protection. She often regulated what we ate, and we were never allowed to eat in other people's houses no matter how close they were related to us.

She did not trust people but also was always very concerned about her children being poisoned or had *juju* (voodoo) applied to harm us.

I stayed in the village for most of the six-week period until school in Navrongo Secondary school reopened in the middle of August 1972.

Before returning from the United States of America, I was still undecided as to which school I wanted to attend to complete my secondary school education (GCE A levels). After several discussions with my family and friends and after considering the transportation cost and other expenses, I decided to go back to my former school because it was a lot closer and I also had an all-expense-paid scholarship and did not want to add to the drain of students that was going on in the Northern part of Ghana to the Southern part as discussed earlier. I had not yet completed some of the reasons why I wanted to attend Navasco..

One item that was foremost when I was in the lower classes was that most of the best students of our school after GCE O levels did not stay back in the Northern and Upper Regional Schools. The bright students were often lured away to attend GCE A-level schools in the southern schools such as Achimota School in Accra, Prempeh College in Kumasi, and Bishop Herman High School in the Volta region of Ghana. These schools were the prestigious schools, and the schools were those that had excellent scores in the West African GCE O-level examination, which was the same examination taken in all countries in the British Commonwealth. The brightest students from the Northern and Upper Regions of the Country leaving to go down south to attend excellent schools was a form of brain drain within the country. The GCE A-level scores were not as good in the north as it was in the south. The northern schools then kept their own meager students or attracted the not-so-bright students from the south. The result of this brain drain was low standards in Navasco and other northern and upper region schools. As a result of the aforementioned reasons only, I stayed in Navasco to complete my A levels (advanced level).

Mr. MacDonald, a British expatriate and mathematics and physics teacher, was the headmaster of Navasco at this time. He was not only an intelligent teacher, but he was also a very dedicated and diligent worker indeed. He worked relentlessly in administering the school and could often be seen driving the school bus or working on the school's tractors to go to the boreholes of the school to fetch water for students' meals to be made. I often admired the headmaster because I could not see how somebody could leave his home country England and come to sacrifice so much for Navasco and its students.

Our own Ghanaian teachers were not even close to such dedication. His work ethic was exemplary which is something I up-to-date still admire and have tried to emulate. We are all still grateful for his hard work and sacrifice to the students of Navasco and to Ghana at large. On the other hand, some Ghanaian teachers who were assigned to northern schools to teach often declined because the northern and upper regions were supposedly too hot for them. Here was a man who was bred and raised in a cold environment who sacrificed himself and whose dedication to people he had no knowledge off till he was brought to teach us was exemplary. Under Mr. McDonald's guidance as headmaster, Navasco expanded tremendously. New dormitories were built, and new programs such as agricultural education were introduced to the forefront of our school's curriculum. The school, which was often considered a poor academic institution, was now made into an academic powerhouse in the whole of Ghana which was one of main goals of wanting to study in Navasco..

After I came back, I was welcomed wholeheartedly by the school, and the academia and managerial leaders of the school were excited to have me back. The school in late 1970 had just undergone a strike. I was not in support of the strike because I did not think the reasons given by the strike leaders were enough to justify a strike. The strike's underpinning reason was over the students not wanting to eat kenkey (dough made from corn). I was amazed as to how some of the student ring leaders were well fed at the end of the school term but when they returned to school after the holidays they mainly looked like skeletons and often looked as if they were suffering from Kwashiokor.. These same students were not grateful for what the school and the government were doing for them. To me the student leaders who were charismatic and had future political aspirations wanted to use deceptive means to get the masses of students from tribes such as the Kassena Nankanis, the Dargartis, and the Kusasis to join them. The leaders were also very ungrateful, and I was not going to participate in the strike. After coming from the United States of America, I even supported my distaste for strikes because as students we did not pay school fees and virtually had everything handed to us on a silver platter that we did not appreciate. America, the most prosperous nation in the world, did not do this to their students. Why weren't we appreciative of everything that we got free? Everybody grew up wanting and demanding everything free without thinking or wanting to know where the monies came from. Also, at this time the discipline in Navasco became very lapsed, and the school had a school dance (disco) band, which began to attract students who were not disciplined and also were not dedicated in their desire for an exceptional education.

Getting a secondary school education seemed to be the goal of most of the students.

I came into the A level (advanced) very well prepared, but I had made up my mind that I was going to go back to the United States to further my education. I was more determined to pursue my goal of being the first person in my family and the Bulbia village to get university education. I had visited University of Wisconsin-Madison and Eau Claire when I was an exchange student a number of times for concerts and also for the forensic student activities and had concluded from what I saw that I would return to attend the university. As a child and pupil, I often heard my father wishing he had the opportunity to go to a university. I took this mantle in that I wanted to be the first person in my family not only to go to a university but also to study medicine. I often accompanied my maternal uncle to the bush to get selective roots and plants for ailments such as headaches, bezoars, abdominal pain; and we made the plant niri to induce labor in pregnant females. I wanted if I became a modern medical doctor to integrate my traditional medicine with "modern" medicine.

In order to encourage me and remind me what my goal was, I wrote "medico" on all my school books, my dormitory room also, and started my quest to meet my final goal.

After the first year of the A level, lower sixth form, elections were to be held for leaders of the students. It was the first time I ever ran politically for any position, and I came up second. The headmaster made me the first chaplain prefect (in charge of school's religious activity) in the school because he knew how dedicated a Catholic I was before my departure for the United States of America.

He was also aware as a person who had grown up in an Islamic religious background that I was the person to choose for this leadership position. I was also made the assistant senior prefect.

The headmaster was not aware of the transformation I had undergone in the United States of America, especially my feelings toward religious personnel whether they were Christians, Moslems and/or Buddhists. I was also a member of the student Council of Navasco.

One aspect that I thought would be helpful to the student and faculty was something I had noticed and remained disturbed about the whole time I was in Navrongo Secondary School. It was the fact that the school's teaching staff lived in separate houses. Here we were demonstrating and talking about the apartheid system in South Africa, and right in our own midst, we had a segregated camp, which we condoned. I passed for the resolution based on my own experience to remove all faculty enclaves based on race, nationality, or tribal affiliation. All Americans stayed within certain designated areas. So were the British we had, and the Ghanaian teachers were also in their own enclave. I thought that by mixing the faculty housing more cohesiveness could be attained. I thought that Americans and the British would like to know us better and understand our culture if they were made to mix with us.

When this resolution was brought up in the student council, a lot of the students and the faculty advisory board were not aware of this, and some actually disagreed only to find out that I was right after I had presented to the council the housing plans.

After having the resolution passed, an attempt was made to carry the resolution through. I had the same silent opposition, and I was not aware whether it was coming from the faculty or from the students. Eventually it was carried out, and we all benefited from it. The faculty interacted more, and the expatriate teachers got to know more about Ghanaians and our culture.

However, everybody was surprised that I was not as religious as I was before going away to the United States. Some attributed it to me growing up, but others attributed it to the fact that I had gone to the United States. I still went to church and made sure that every student understood their role and their importance to the school and the country at large. One of the conflicts I had was during the Ramadan period. Some of the Moslem students wanted to be excused from school activities because they were fasting. They were often late to school activities, and since the senior prefect was a Moslem, they felt they were in the privileged group. I, however, objected to any special deals using the Ramadan to break institutional laws. My mother, in so far as I have ever known her, never used the fasting period as an excuse during this atonement period not to carry out her religious or nonreligious responsibilities. One is not supposed to make excuses or want to be treated differently or be excused from school functions. My mother still went to farm and did not curtail duty and responsibilities during the fasting period. She did not use the Ramadan period, which is a period of atonement, as an excuse to neglect responsibilities. Some of the Moslem students who were Dagombas were furious, but I refused to relent. They could not accuse me of not being familiar with the religion, and I demanded nothing different from the Christians during their holidays or fasting periods. I was born and grew up in the Islam religion, which was used to mold me as a child, and I owe my health to it.

During my first year in my GCE A level, I studied physics, chemistry, and biology; and I started applying to schools especially in the United States because I had an American high school diploma and excellent GCE O-level examination scores. I applied to the University of Wisconsin-Eau Claire mainly because I had personally been to the school and also because it was close to my American parents in Bloomer, Wisconsin.

I got admitted to University of Wisconsin-Eau Claire in my first year in lower sixth form in Navrongo Secondary School. Knowing that I already had admission to the University of Wisconsin took a lot of pressure off me because I did not want to stay in Ghana for my university education.

I studied but not as seriously as I could. I had also applied for a scholarship by the Ghana government to study veterinary or human medicine.

The rest of the years in Navrongo Secondary School was uneventful, and the years passed by rather quickly.

The headmaster of Navrongo was very helpful to me obtaining a Ghana government scholarship.

At the end of the year, the headmaster wished me the best, and I went home at the end of the school year. I left Navasco knowing that I had fulfilled all the reasons I had to go to Navasco. I had in my own way succeeded academically and by competing with others directly or indirectly had brought Navasco's academic standing a lot higher than it was when I first went there. The village boy from Bulbia along with now Dr. Gyesika Agambila helped to put Navasco's name locally and internationally. Navasco then became an institution that younger intelligent northern boys and girls looked up to get an excellent education. Navasco became a household name and not just the institution of sports. I felt that I had played my part to also uplift the importance of education in a society that had grabbed to the notion that Western education had evil intentions and was meant to destroy our proud African culture. I therefore went home to arrange to travel back to the United States of America to study at the University Wisconsin-Eau Claire. My father was also very proud that what he could not do was being done by his son.

As a farewell tour, I stayed again with my junior brother in Tamale.

After a visit to my brother in Tamale, I went back to Bulbia to say goodbye to my parents and especially to my maternal grandmother to whom I was very close to. I explained to Grandma Amina that I was going back to the United States of America to study further. She looked up to me even though she was blind and said, "Nyaba, why is it that your younger brother is working and sending me money and you keep failing and failing in school? The schools will be fed up with you because you are taking too long to finish your schooling. Nyaba, with all your big head, you want to tell me that you do not have brains?" mockingly said my grandma. My grandmother equated my going from school to school as a demotion, and she concluded that my junior brother was more intelligent than I am; that's why he was working and making money, and I was still going to school penniless.

After I explained to my grandmother that it was at a higher level of study, she potentially understood me.

Something that struck me right in the chest like a bullet was when my grandmother told me that if I went on this trip, I was not going to come back and see her alive. All of a sudden, I became saddened and sat by my grandmother to explain to her.

After I explained to her my desire to be a medical doctor, she became more enlightened because she thought it was an honorable profession as was a fetish priest (traditional healer) in our village. I did not refrain from talking to my grandmother about my travel plans.

Somehow after my grandmother brought out this idea that I was not going to come back to see her alive, I began to spend more time with her to understand certain items that had perplexed me about my maternal grandmother.

Since I grew up to become aware, my maternal grandmother was blind. Based on how well my grandmother knew her environment especially her surroundings and the position of her water pots and other belongings, I concluded that my grandmother's blindness was a gradual process rather than an acute process. I was very curious to know why she was blind.

My mother was very uncomfortable and always brushed me off. She told me that my grandmother got blind from a venomous viper spitting into her eyes and making her blind.

Still I was more curious; but questions to my mother, maternal aunts, and uncles almost always fell on deaf ears. This was an opportune time for me to have an extended time with my grandmother. My grandmother described a period of gradual loss of her eyesight and how it was associated with nervousness and a sudden onset of progressive darkness to total blindness.

She also thought that it had something to do with a *kpaka*, a lump on her anterior neck. I often saw a protuberance on her left lateral neck region on my grandmother's neck, but I was afraid to ask questions, and neither she nor my mother volunteered any answers. At that time children were not allowed to ask questions that had to do with somebody's privacy. It was in medical school that I gradually began to put things together to figure out that my grandmother probably got blind from hyperthyroidism (Grave's disease) or toxic thyrotoxicosis.

The day I left Bulbia for Accra to pursue my long and winding road for the rest of my life, I went to Grandma to extend my goodbye wishes because as she had earlier told me, I was almost sure I was not going to come back to see her again. I went back to my mother and started to cry. My grandmother wanted to pray, but as in our Kantonsi-Mamprusi tradition, a woman would not lead in prayer to our ancestors and deities; so she called my oldest maternal uncle (Njahaba Kpanbinaba) to carry out the task. Libation was poured, and a hen was sacrificed for our ancestors and deities. In the supine position, the hen landed, which meant that our prayers were accepted and blessed by our god, deities, and ancestors. Had the sacrificed hen landed in the prone position, that would have been translated as rejection of our sacrifice to our ancestors and deities of our village.

The libation was performed, and the hen was sacrificed for my ancestors and deities to guard me to the land of the unknown. I went back to my parents and enjoyed talking to my sisters. I ended up falling asleep rather late and got up early in order to walk back to Walewale, which is still a journey of about twelve miles and a distance to reckon with; but this time I was not barefooted, and the heat of the sun was not that severe or intense.

From Walewale, I passed to Tamale to say goodbye to my younger brother who was by then working for Ghana Airways as the station assistant in Tamale. The following day I left by bus to Accra. When in Accra, we went to see some of the present and former AFS students and members. I met some of those who had gone a year before I did. A good friend of mine came toward me and asked me what I was going to the United States of America to study. I told him that it was my ambition to study medicine. He immediately walked back twice and asked me if I were dreaming. I was immediately taken aback and amazed at his reaction and response. "The U.S. is not a place for a black man to study medicine since they have strict qualifications required, and on top of that, none of your parents are doctors," he said. "How did you think you can get into medical school in the USA?" he said rather loudly and discouragingly.

He told me to continue to dream. All of a sudden, I said one more time that I was going to the United States to do medicine, and it will be done no matter the obstacles that lay before me.

I promised him that he will be the first person I will visit when I completed my medical education and come back home.

After a short period of stay in Accra, I left for the United States to begin my education and muscle my way through a long route of trials and minimal errors.

At this time the changes in Ghana from a right-hand-driving nation to the left-hand-drive format (*onifa, onifa*) had just began in 1974, and I found it was an opportune time to initiate a new step in my life by entering into the second stage of a cripple's life. Everything is possible. Who expected a young man to come from his hut in Bulbia to become one of the chosen few to represent their country and also attain one of the best secondary school scores in the country? The only person I thought who could defeat me at this time was myself, and I was not in any way going to let that happen.

THIRD PHASE OF ZARA'S CRIPPLED SON

University Education (undergraduate and graduate) in America and my maternal grandmother Amina's funeral.

I n August 1974 I returned to the United States of America to study at the University of Wisconsin-Eau Claire. When I came into Eau Claire, I stayed with my American family in Bloomer, Wisconsin. About a week after my arrival and stay in Bloomer, I left Bloomer for Eau Claire to start my university education.

Again the weather was very cold for us Africans. I got to meet other African students in the university. My first year was very lonely but rather uneventful. I made a lot of friends, both American and foreign students. I participated in intramural soccer and volleyball and enjoyed participating. At this time in the United States, soccer was not a popular sport. It was mainly played by the international students who included students from Nigeria, Kenya, Greece, Colombia, Argentina, and Ghana.

During the holiday periods, we had no other place to go, and a lot of the foreign students could not afford to travel back to our countries to spend our holidays.

Since we had no place to go to during the holidays, we often moved from dormitory to dormitory. The holiday periods were the loneliest times for a foreign student especially during summer breaks.

My university education in Wisconsin was very, very interesting in several aspects. In the dormitories, we the African students came to realize that whenever a black student was placed in a room with a white student, one could predict that about ninety-nine percent of the time the white students never showed up. Initially we could not explain why it was happening until I became a resident assistant. I was one of the first black resident assistants in the University of Wisconsin-Eau Claire in the history of the university. During my tenure as a resident assistant in Towers Hall, students did not show up for their assigned rooms in my assigned dormitory.

It affected some of the sensitive African students. After discussions with other African students, we could not blame ourselves in any way, but we learnt how to share rooms and accommodate some of our colleagues who could not afford accommodation on or off campus at this time. We were beginning to realize a different America for what I had experienced in Bloomer, Wisconsin, as an exchange student.

After several attempts of trying to get an apartment had failed, we all resigned to the fact that the university dormitories were where we belonged to, even though they were more expensive for our budget. They were also much safer and exposed us less to the elements of racial divide. Even in the classes, it was rather strange. In our school system, we often shared our learning or note writing with each other. The brilliant students had no qualms helping the non-intelligent students. However, in the University of Wisconsin in those days it was almost a taboo for a minority student to ask the white students for help especially when one was absent from class for one reason or the other.

All the African students and minority students felt that there was some bias in the grading system. One could not understand how two students who worked on the same project and experiment and came out with the same conclusion could come up with varying scores, sometimes two-grade-point difference. Some of the white students did see some of the injustices and unfairness and often made complaints on our behalf to no concern of the professors.

The senior minority students often also directed younger students which professors to avoid.

Most of the African and black students in our discussions often decided just to study to get by because we knew beforehand that no matter how hard one studied, one could barely do better than a B grade. We beforehand had been warned by our senior students on this issue, so we were more than prepared when the issue started arising.

This was an experience with all the African students even in other schools in the university system. The South African students and Chinese students were loved by the chemistry and physics department. I often discussed how they got research assistantship when we had all applied. In some cases I was told that it was part of their financial aid package. However, we often joked among ourselves that for an equally brilliant African or black student, I was not likely to get a research position because of innate bias in the department of certain races.

In my days in UW-Eau Claire, the class that was a taboo was the genetics class, which was known to have had the fewest African or black students taking the course and nobody could get better than a C grade. It was indeed a hostile environment. The professor was baldheaded because when he grew his hair, it was curly and kinky like a Negro, which he very much resented. In one of our self-counseling services, we indicated that if a professor had such negativity about one's genetics, it was no wonder that such inferior thoughts could be carried to harm innocent persons. The students (African and black) students often acted as our own counselors. The older students were often counselled the juniors about what classes to take because the school-assigned counselors would often advise us to take courses outside the programs we wanted to graduate in. "The chemistry class will be too difficult for you coming from Africa. Why don't you take this history class?" said one of my assigned advisors. That was the first and only time I ever spoke to her until I graduated with a bachelor's degree in chemistry. We had students who were advised by counselors who had enough credits to graduate but could not be assigned to a program, and we made sure it did not happen to us.

The university's programs did not encourage any unison between the American black students and the foreign black students. A lot of us were wise enough to realize this and did all we could to initiate programs such as parties and foreign student programs to help integrate the groups.

Our experience in the school with regard to race relations was the same as what we experienced when we tried to rent or intermingle with the Eau Claire community. There was innate fear of the Negroid male figure.

At times we the foreign black students were more "accepted" than the American black students. As foreign black students, we were often thought as transients and were not going to be a permanent fixture of the American society.

African student parties were often spectacular. It was a time we could forget our frustrations and loneliness, and we could express our experiences together.

The predominant groups were Nigerian students. The Nigerian students flaunted their wealth because their country was one of the richest if not the richest in the continent of Africa at that time, and the students definitely showed it. They attracted more females and other students with their wealth or presumed wealth. Whilst the rest of the African students were struggling to get money to eat, some students were driving Mercedes-Benz cars in school and often stood up in the crowd as rich students whose parents were chiefs and kings in Africa.

The other students often wondered. Whilst the rest of African students were struggling to get money to eat and pay their school fees, others often flaunted their wealth or presumed wealth in parties in order to attract beautiful women.

Whilst the rest of the African students were struggling to get money to buy books, some students drove Mercedes-Benzes and other expensive cars in school. We often wondered how rich these students were. What was interesting was that the same students driving these expensive cars were often the same students who could not pay their school fees at the beginning or end of the semester or academic year. African parties were often like a United Nations General Assembly gathering, and they made us for once not think of the numerous problems we had in adjusting in a society, which had no respect for strangers who came to this country mainly to get an education. It was generally a worthwhile project even with all the difficulties we had to go through. We learnt about how to get along well with people who would not necessarily invite you to dinner or who wished bad things could happen to us. I stayed throughout my University of Wisconsin experience in Eau Claire in the dormitory. During the holidays we worked on campus cleaning the dormitories, toilets, and classes in preparation for the next semester. Some of the foreign students felt they would not clean toilets because it was an undignified work for university students. Those of us who had no money did, and from there we had extra monies for things that were not covered in our scholarship programs.

The loneliest time of my university education was during the holidays when everybody was going home to see their parents and siblings and all I could do was to move from one dormitory room to the next. I often cried during these periods because I was lonely and missed my parents and siblings. I never could imagine that I could miss my siblings at all when I was leaving. During the day or nighttime of the holidays, one could hear my local Mamprusi music blasting whilst I sang 'Tosi Yuma'(local Mamprusi songs) to myself and danced till I got tired and went to sleep. I often heard my mother talking to me and touching me, and I got up the next day refreshed and found a new air of strength to continue my education.

Initially I would go to visit my American host family, but to my surprise on one Saturday they marched to my dormitory, and my American host dad came in angrily to tell me I was no longer welcomed to their house. I sat down on several occasions to learn or understand what happened that brought such an action. I had done nothing to them to warrant such a reaction since I respected my American parents fully and did not expect such behavior. Several entities came through my mind. I was very much set with what I wanted to achieve and where I wanted to be in the future, and I was always very cautious with what I said or I did. I had my circle of friends whose association I adored. My American host father was curious that I was too ambitious, and he could not understand why I wanted to go into medicine when my parents were so poor. I refrained from discussing my future plans and other issues of African poverty and the role donations were being made on behalf of African people because at times I had different opinions that people did not want to hear or know. To Americans every African grew up poor, malnourished, and helpless. Growing up in my village and surrounding areas, we never really had a definition for poverty. All children ran around naked and had no shoes, which we attributed to the weather; and yes, some houses could provide three square meals a day when others could not. There was not much difference, and we were happy and secure. Nobody was afraid to play outside in fear of being kidnapped; nobody was afraid of being sexually molested or being shot. The environment was peaceful, and that was more important to our families. It was when I went down south of Ghana that I began to notice some difference in the quality of life, but the happiness of life did not equate to material possessions.

At this time of my life, I did not like to be discouraged by other people who underestimated my desire to become a medical doctor.

After this episode with my American parents, I was rather strengthened and learnt to be alone and began to distrust people but became more intent on attaining my goal. I got more involved with my fellow African students and did not travel outside the town of Eau Claire during the holidays. Along with other African and international students, we played soccer, which was at that time not a popular sport in this country. After also going through what I and other African or Negroid students went through in the university, I became more involved in efforts to end the apartheid system in South Africa at that time. At times I had conflicting views about what the apartheid system really was. On one hand I thought that during the apartheid or segregation period in the United States and now in South Africa, black people learnt to depend on themselves. There were black high schools, black colleges, black professional teams, and black musicians. The youth were taught by the best, because most black teachers had no choice but to share their knowledge and expertise to their own. Great schools like the Tuskegee Institute, Spellman College, Howard University, and the Hampton College could not have existed if blacks had the luxury of being able to attend or teach in white schools. There was a certain expectation. The only disadvantage was the mental slavery segregation brought. If one could live in a system in which one could be with his or her kind, like wild animals do but yet respect each other, we as children of God could live separately, respect each other and still have equal rights. Animals and other creatures of the earth live segregated lives, protect themselves but still do understand their role in protecting their ecosystem. In America, because of segregation a number of very good secondary schools and universities were nurtured and taught by very well-trained African American teachers and professors who could not get work at the all-white schools. What happened in America was that as soon as desegregation was instituted, most of the fabric of the African American school system went into disarray, and students bore the brunt of being bused to desegregate schools. What this also caused was to also disintegrate the African American family unit and schools and went a long way to destroy the family unit and proud education the African American had at that time. The black students were then left in the public school systems where the best teachers never wanted to go; the students lost confidence in their teachers, and the teachers in turn only saw teaching as a means of an income and not a passion and desire to educate young men and women to become the best. This turn of events has resulted in the continued decay of public education to the deplorable state we see it today.

Most whites who did not want their children to go to school with other minorities simply enrolled their children in private schools that were out of reach to the average African American. This resulted in a decrease in the quality of education in the African American society. Children spent more hours riding buses to meet Supreme Court rules and less time studying. Children had more time to interact on ill-defined plans in the absence of the unit family in the bus resulting in crimes and other uncalled-for activities, which are not condoned by this society. After noticing this trend that ending segregation took something out of the black man. It took his pride and entrepreneurship and knocked out the most important cornerstone of a family: the male. The black man became the pillar of hatred, and an avenue had to be created in order to keep him still in bondage. Instead of creating new and modern schools, prisons were created in order to curtail the black man's political and entrepreneurial spirit. Students in public schools were made to follow such liberal rules by organizations that did not allow the same rules in their communities. School uniform—which was a form of equality, pride, and stability—began to be assaulted and destroyed. Children could wear whatever they wanted. Since there was no dress code for the schools, there was no defined disciplinary rules for children to follow. The public school systems have gradually became prison or security institutions because of indiscipline and people fighting frustration created by the generation before. Teachers who were seen as the extension of the family began to be afraid of the young men and women they were to teach and care for. They began to be afraid of their own students and children in school. The grading system failed, and learning became nonexistent because social promotion became the norm resulting in the loss of a generation of the youth who would have shepherded us into the next millennium.

After observing and experiencing these observations at times, I felt the South African system should be left alone so that South African blacks could dignify themselves. In my mind I felt that the system could indicate that all humans were born equal and that all humans are the same in the eyes of the Almighty and all races could be proud of who they were. This could involve upgrading schools, transportation, and educational principles in all provinces and putting up programs to encourage the black South Africans to gradually come to the level of all South Africans be they white, mulatto, or others. I still felt that ending apartheid was not going to make a dent in maintaining human dignity since humans will always find another way to distinguish themselves; but the potential of producing a big class system, which we would bring in a new form of inequality where only the few elite blacks, mulattos, or whites or well-to-do South Africans could change the white powerhouse. On the other hand, no matter what I thought, it still involved bringing awareness to the human plight to this country, which had gone through and is still undergoing such experience. I went around and participated in all aspects of the resistance in South Africa. In my small ways I refused to use certain banks and even refused to drink beverages that had companies dealing with South Africa. Even though I was a poor student and struggling at that time, I still wanted to participate. I also joined in some of the boycotts that were organized by Mr. Gene Robinson and the Pan-African movement. I had different ideas as to what kind of South Africa I wanted to evolve, and even though it was not a popular one and I could be seen by some people as being a black segregationist, I was still willing to listen to all sides and in my small way bring the evil of one being made to feel inferior and degraded by a fellow human being who had the same color of blood and who would end up being devoured by the same ecosystem that encompasses the world. This became one of my lifelong passions. I want to see South

Africa liberated in my lifetime as seen in above documentation that I made during one of my solemn moments in my life. Liberation by itself means nothing without the economic security that has evaded the black race the longest.

I also started to learn how to drive in my second year in college. My friends often laughed at me because I had never driven a car before. Indeed I was excited as the driver's education came through the school, and I was proud to write home and inform my family about it. Letter writing became my main mode of communication. At the time I had to book a telephone call in the post office for about four weeks in advance in order to get a telephone call through to Ghana unlike today when calls can be made anytime directly from my village, Bulbia. I hardly used this method of communication because it often made me more homesick whenever I heard my mother's voice. In those days in emergencies a telegraph was often sent to me especially when my grandmother died.

The saddest moment of my life come in September 1977 when I got a telegram telling me that my beloved grandmother (maternal) had died. I did not eat for days and wept because I could hear my grandmother telling me that I was not going back to see her alive. I cried and called my fellow international students to pray in memory of my grandmother, and we did. "Your grandmother is with Allah and your ancestors," said one of my friends. In the Kantonsi micronation, when a grandmother or grandparent dies, it is a time of celebration by the grandchildren and not a mourning period. I tried to enable myself to think that way, but it was not easy.

After my friends consoled me and said a prayer with me, I went into the room; and for the first time that I would remember, I poured libation by putting some Bisquick powder in water and offered it to my grandmother and our Kantonsi dieties.. I suddenly felt better but could not be myself until I went for the funeral, which was yet to come. My grandmother had made me promise to her that no matter where I was, I would attend her funeral when she died.

As if my grandmother Amina's death inspired me, I applied and became a resident assistant in the Towers Hall of the University of Wisconsin-Eau Claire, and it did become a challenge but an experience that has helped me up-to-date.

I was made a resident assistant, one of the first African resident assistants in the school. My duties included counseling students or others ranging from homesickness and loneliness to more mundane situations such as depression and dating problems. I again also got to see more racial problems in my one year and final year of my undergraduate studies.

There were families who did not want their children to be in my hall. They never told me why, but I could sense the reason. At this point of my life, I started paying less attention to racial issues because some of the issues I dealt with were rather pathetic. Many younger students in and outside my hall also approached me with their problems, and those I could not help I often referred for expert assistance. I enjoyed my senior year both academically and socially. I participated in several extracurricular activities, but along the way, I seriously started thinking about my desire to be a doctor. As a pre–medical student, nobody encouraged me. People including university counselors often discouraged me, but I was confident that I had not studied to my capability. Why did I have to study so hard in an atmosphere where no matter how hard I worked, I was always guaranteed a lower grade than the average white student? Some counselors often told me how it was impossible to make it to medical school without any family member being in the profession and also not being a citizen of the United State of America.

I was also not sure how the system worked, so after completing my undergraduate work in three years, I decided to go into graduate school to start my graduate studies in biochemistry. I was admitted to the graduate chemistry programs in the University of Cincinnati and University of Wisconsin-Milwaukee.

In the fall of 1977 I entered into the graduate chemistry program at the University of Wisconsin-Milwaukee. It was in this program that my intensity and level of interest in medicine began to peak. I was a graduate teaching assistant, and I taught undergraduate chemistry programs. I loved teaching, and I motivated a lot of black students to study. I taught a chemistry class, which was a prerequisite to enter into the school of nursing program. The first year I had a lot of international and black students who did exceptionally well. A lot of the students expressed that I motivated them. The following semester

I had no single African American student in the same class, and this continued till I left the program for medical school education.

In 1978 I decided it was time to go home most importantly to pay my homage to my deceased grandmother. It was the first anniversary of her death. In the Kantonsi tribe, we have the seven-day ceremony followed by a forty-day mourning period, and the last ceremony is usually a year after the death of an elderly person. When a grandparent dies, the mourning period is usually staged by the grandchildren. The grandchildren generally carry a *kun la* (a calabash with a white cloth), which is carried by the oldest grandchild and carried all over the village announcing the death of the grandparent. The white cloth or sheet in the calabash is part of the burial white cloth, which is used to wrap the deceased body before burial. In the Kantonsi tribe, burials take place within twenty-four hours after the person is declared officially dead. The belief is that the spirit has already left the body onto the next incarnation period of the next world. Kantonsis believe that all of us incarnate as lizards. The calabash (*kun la*) becomes the center of attention of the funeral. During the funeral, I wept, but I was quickly stopped by my uncles. They encouraged me not to mourn my grandmother's death by crying because as a grandchild I am supposed to celebrate my grandmother's good life that she had on this earth and to ask God and our ancestors to receive her soul and accept it in the next world.

The third day a dance called *jugu*, which is a special dance only performed during the funeral of a grandparent and nobody else, was organized and carried out.

The Kantonsi tribe believe that jugu songs should not be sung outside a funeral; otherwise, some immediate family member was going to be called to join our ancestors in the next world. There were times when I was a child when I would imitate one of the songs of jugu in the house. My mother would usually quickly come to close my mouth or call out for me to stop the practice. "Do you want somebody in the family to die?" she would often protest.

I also learnt that one does not keep and expose photographs of the deceased because that is an invitation for your grandparent's spirit not to be accepted for the next world.

Jugu dancing was carried out. Songs of praises were heaped on my grandmother. I participated in the dancing, and we danced all night to the next morning.

In the midst of the dance, a grandchild, not necessarily the oldest, often carried the kun la, which rotates in rhythmic fashion on top of the middle of the head. It is very mystical as one has to hold the kun la in the position rather tightly so that the calabash does not fall and break. If it falls, it means a curse to the living family members or a natural disaster is set to take place. The subsequent days I realized that I had no place to go but sit down and talk like I did with my grandmother, and it made me very sad and lonely. It is also customary after the funeral ceremonies to go from house to house to thank every household for their help and appreciation of their roles in the funeral process.

In the Mamprusi and Kantonsis who are both members of the Mole-Dagbani heritage, the tribal system divides activities into family units all to serve the village or villages. The groups often includes *nanchina* (head of the young people), *akara* (the head of council of elders of the village, *lunsi na* (the family in charge of drumming and the drums of the village), and *kumdu* (the household responsible for the digging of the graves for burial). Every household has a responsibility to play in the community, and they take that responsibility seriously without any desire to be compensated or paid, and it is the responsibility of the grandchildren to make sure it is safe. In the first week everybody sits outside on mats called *zana* mats, and prayers (Islamic) are said, and sacrifices to our deities are also made. Women are not allowed to sit in the *soagri* (a shade made to protect people from the sun and often used as a gathering center) with the men but are required to be in the compound of the dead.

If there is a male spouse, he sits outside with the other chief mourners most of the time for the first week, and then after the week the forty-day period continues. On the other hand, a group of women sits in the dead person's room till the end of the forty-day period. By the time I went home, I could not participate in these ceremonies.

I got to the village after arriving in Accra very quickly because I was very emotional. When I got home, my mother had already prepared for my return. I rested that first day, and after two days all the activities to celebrate my grandmother's life began.

Whilst fulfilling my graduate chemistry education and teaching, I was also applying to medical schools knowing that I did not have the right visas for the programs. A friend of mine from Nigeria, Joy Ogolo, brought to my attention about St. George's University School of Medicine, and she encouraged me to apply to the school. This school, she told me, was located in the Caribbean Sea and would require me to leave the United States and go to Grenada to acquire a medical education. I thought it was her way to get rid of me since she knew I was interested in her as a girlfriend. I applied after I took the MCAT (medical college aptitude test), and lo and behold, I was accepted. I continued my graduate chemistry and biochemistry program, but all at his time my main interest was in medicine and not as a graduate student in chemistry. Teaching chemistry was a lot of fun, and I enjoyed teaching even though l did not have a long-term desire to continue to teach.

After several months after applying to several schools, I one day got a thick letter from Bay Shore, New York. This letter was delivered to me through my friend Ms. Joy Ogolo. When I opened it up, it was an acceptance letter; I screamed and started to jump around. I could not believe it that I had been accepted. I went to Bay Shore, New York, for an interview to the school. On this two-day trip, I was very exhausted.

I was determined to leave the United States of America to go anywhere in the world for a chance to study medicine. Most of my friends and schoolmates did all they could to discourage me from going to this school. I had no single friend who supported me. My final decision was made when I made a call to the Ghana embassy to inquire about my scholarship. I spoke to the education director who told me a little about Grenada and also said that the Ghana government could not afford to give me a scholarship to go to a medical school in this country because it was too expensive. He told me the school fees in St. George's University School of Medicine were affordable. After speaking to the director, I made up the rest of my mind that I was going to Grenada. I had an opportunity to study medicine toward which I have been working hard to achieve since I was a child.

Zara's crippled child who had undergone all medical efforts to get him to walk was determined to go to medical school and become a physician to help other people who were in the same predicament as I was.

In order not to have more discouraging news from my friends, I remained very quiet and continued to teach chemistry as a graduate teaching assistant. I enjoyed teaching very much, and since my father was a teacher, I did not have any problems expressing myself in crowds.

I decided not to call my parents because I had contacted my junior brother, and his response was not very encouraging. "You just want to get the name doctor on your name, don't you?" said my brother. He then added, "I advise you not to leave the United States and go to another country"; he reiterated in a letter to me. I did not respond to my brother's letter and only responded to his letter after I had enrolled in St. George's University School of Medicine in St. George's, Grenada in August of 1979. I did not have much space after buying my school books and other necessities of life. I made all my flight arrangements and left Milwaukee rather quietly and unceremoniously and made my way to New York City en route to St. George's, Grenada, in August 1979, and this began the most important phase of my life.

The making of Zara's Crippled Son as a Medical doctor and life in the West Indies as a medical student.

In August 1979 I flew out of JFK Airport in New York City for the Caribbean island of Grenada. I did not know much about the Caribbean; but I knew of important people such as L'ouverture of Haiti, Codjo of Jamaica, Nana of Jamaica, and many other slaves and the struggles they went through in slave ships while bound in chains. How could it be so bad if great people who were possibly my ancestors from the Kantonsi tribe had gone through these oceans chained and bound and yet they made it? How couldn't I make it when I was traveling on a plane in my own free will? I thought and thought and could not remove the thoughts from my mind. It gave me an incentive to let me know I was doing the right thing. In the plane I had no idea what was going to happen, but I was determined to succeed no matter what lay in front or back of me. The weight of my decision to leave the United States of America did not fall on my shoulders until the American Airlines plane took off from the airport.

As the plane took off, I clasped my hands and said my prayer to every god, deity, and my ancestors especially my grandmother Amina whose funeral I had last flown to attend a year before.

I wanted all my ancestors to guard me because I was out to do something that I loved and something I was the first in my family to do. I got the window side of the plane and felt lonely but secure all of a sudden. I was not accompanied to the airport by anybody or relative. I missed when my mother would carry my luggage from Bulbia to Walewale to see me off to school. She could often enchant her prayers and exultations to our ancestors and Allah to guard and protect me. Every thought of my mind would come flowing. I asked myself several questions and went ahead and answered them to my own satisfaction. There were other passengers on board with me, but I did not say much and did not seem to know or care that they existed.

After several hours flying, the plane arrived in Bridgetown, Barbados, in the Caribbean. I got off and took my luggage and went to the side of Liat (the Caribbean local airlines) where I was to board for the rest of the journey to Grenada.

This plane, unlike the first by American Airlines, was very small, and it was the first time that other students who were taking the same risk I was were present. I was so nervous that I could not carry on any conversations on the plane, and I held on tight to the seat in front of me. The plane tossed all over the place. I kept tossing from place to place even with a seatbelt on; and the more the wind blew, the more I feared I was going to join my grandmother in the deep Caribbean Sea.

On approach to the Grenada Airport, the plane suddenly dropped a more than tolerable distance toward the ground. I grabbed onto my seat and anything I could get hold off as tightly as I could. The plane finally landed, and there began a more-than-exciting life in the island of Grenada or, as we know it, the Spice Isles or Nutmeg Country.

Along with two other students, we chartered a taxi to take us to St. George's where the school was located. The road from Grandville to St. George's was a narrowing and winding one with several potholes. The driver kept trying to evade the potholes; but the more he did, the scarier the ride to the school got. We had no seatbelts, so we kept rolling around with our luggage on the seats.

At about 6:00 p.m. we arrived at the University in Grand Anse, Grenada, and then to True Blue where all the freshmen medical students were to stay in the dormitory.

When we arrived, I was so tired that I fell asleep almost immediately after getting some beddings out.

The next day students began to stream in, and I met a few African students. The majority of the students were Americans followed by Nigerians who made up the majority of the black students. I was the only Ghanaian, and we had students from South Africa, Cameroon, and a few North African countries. Before classes started, we familiarized ourselves with the school's surroundings and the second campus in Grand Anse, Grenada, a suburb of St. George's, the capital city and economic center of the people of Grenada.

We often took the local transport buses to town. In Grenada it was very interesting in that the local people who were predominantly of the Negroid race did not expect black students to attend the school. This became evident when we had intramural soccer games in the island. Whenever we had a soccer match, we used the Tanteen football field or the national stadium near St. John's District. During these games, Grenadians almost always saw all the African and a few Grenadian students play on one side and all the white students were on the opposite team.

We the black students were often taken as Grenadians.

One time whilst we were playing a game in St. George's, somebody asked who the teams playing were. A local Grenadian said that it was a game between the dock workers and St. George's University. Some of the black students took this as an insult, but I did not care, and I actually felt that the local people felt that we were part of them, and they cheered and encouraged us to beat our other school team that consisted of all-white students.

Henceforth, our university soccer team was called the dockworkers football team. The first year was generally uneventful, and I enjoyed all the courses that were presented before us.

I also made friends, both white and black; but the school, even though it was in a black country, still had the same racial divide as I experienced in the mainland United States of America, which was rather surprising because I expected intelligent and highly educated people to be broad minded and sensitive to other people's feelings. In fact, what I found out was that as people became more educated, they became more prejudiced or resentful to groups who appeared to threaten their importance. Most of the students were children of medical doctors or other highly educated persons. It seemed to me to be more economic or presumed economic prejudice than of racial prejudice. Students were more comfortable with whoever they wanted to be with, and this seemed to gravitate toward racial preference. For example, in the university, Africans tended to hang together even though our tribal affiliations were far diverse and different. In the cafeteria blacks grouped with each other and whites were often to themselves. Peer pressure also often pushes this type of behavior, and if one violated that divide, oftentimes one would be called a white lover or black lover.

At times I often did not see anything wrong with it as long as we were not forcing people to implement the divide. Both groups of students had the same goal in mind even though their social agenda seemed far wide prejudicial at times.

The school authorities did not encourage each side to break the naturally created racial blocks and in some ways encouraged it to flourish. The school was classified as American citizens pitched against noncitizens. Students were chosen for rotations, externship, or internship from a divisive climate.

At the end of the semester, we had a school break, and most people traveled back to the United States to see their families. Most of the African students or people like me who either could not afford to travel or did not want to stayed back and rested in preparation for the next semester. The following semester we began to get teachers from the continental United States of America for various courses including biochemistry, histology, and anatomy. We formed study groups, and I was responsible for leading the group in biochemistry. Things were generally uneventful. There was no new food for me to adjust to since most of the campus meals were made of American food, and the local food was no different from mine in Bulbia, Ghana.

When our courses began to sound serious enough and I realized I was indeed in a medical school, I got into a shell and did not do much interaction with other students outside our study group.

I moved out of the school-designated dormitories and rented an apartment in Tanteen, near St. George's. In Tanteen with my Nigerian roommate we realized that we were shielded from the Grenada populace since we barely went downtown. As nonboarding students, we were no longer shielded from getting to know the people of Grenada, and life became much better. I met some of the most decent and honorable human beings in the world.

During this time my allowance were not getting to me, so it was one of the lowest period because I had no money. Even though I had no money, one would not really get to know because as an African, the Rastafarians who consider Emperor Haile Selassie as the direct descendant of Judah in Ethiopia made sure we the African students were well stocked with food. They invited us to their farms up in Sauteres; and up the hills and whenever we came back from the farms, we had enough yams, bread, fruit, and plantain to cook and feed ourselves. As an African, I was very grateful for the hospitality these persons of humble living; they gave us things they could have used. They were very much interested in knowing more of Africa, and we were often delighted to share our knowledge with them. Because of the hospitality the Rastaffarians extended to us and because of my teaching experience, I volunteered to teach the advance-level chemistry in the St. George's Government Secondary School in Tanteen. So apart from my studies in the medical school, I volunteered to teach A-level chemistry in the secondary school, which was just a stone's throw from my rented apartment. I enjoyed teaching from my experience as a graduate teaching assistant of the University of Wisconsin-Milwaukee. There was a need for this service since they had no qualified teachers to undertake the task. I willingly volunteered to teach, and it was obvious from the attendance to the class that the students appreciated my teaching. I was very grateful to Grenadians for taking me as part of them.

At the end of the medical school education in Grenada, I got to know every section of Grenada including visits to the Obiah lady in St. Patrick and Tivoli.

At the end of the second year when school closed, everybody left the island including my apartment mate, and I was left alone; so I decided to volunteer in the St. George's General Hospital during the vocation period since I had no place to go. The only place I wanted to go was to go to Ghana to see my parents and siblings and personally inform them that I was a medical student, but I had no money to travel, so I stayed back. I went on medical rounds with some of the British doctors who were the visiting consultants in the hospital.

I had just started some rudimentary clinical medicine in school during the semester, and by not traveling during the holidays, I spent my time doing clinical and voluntary work in the Grenada General Hospital and other chores to help the hospital and the country at large. This holiday period gave me a head start in the clinical portion of my medical education, and it helped shape my ability to work under situations without the technology we have in America. During the holidays, I also got to know the island and its people much better. I went to most of the significant towns such as Tivoli, Sauteres, Petit Martinique, Carriacou, St. John's, and Granville and drove to almost all corners of the island of Grenada.

I also visited the obeah lady, which is an equivalent to the "juju man" or fetish priest in our villages in Ghana. Females played a critical role of treating people from a traditional medicine point of view unlike in my village and other African communities, where it is often played by men. The Rastafarian religion, which I had read about, was fascinating, and the Rastafarians I met made me know that I was special and made me feel at home. In most of the clinics I later headed some clinic programs about, Rastafarian diet that commonly resulted in the development of sub-acute degeneration of the spinal cord because of their strictly vegetarian diet resulting in vitamin B12 deficiency. I went into farms, which were owned by the Rastafarians in the highlands of Grenada, with my friend "Boyo" Thomas. The same form of subsistent farming also existed in Grenada, and the similarity in farming with farming in Ghana was remarkable and made my stay in Grenada an ever-satisfying experience.

I often shared the history and stories of Africa in general and Ghana in particular with the Rastafarians who paid much attention to what I was saying most of the time. My friend "Boyo" Thomas, whom I consider the best friend I have ever had, was a World Cup football player, and I participated playing in football even though I was nowhere near the caliber of Boyo.

During the beginning of the third year, we were moved to the island of St. Vincent where the clinical program was to continue. Leaving Grenada was one of the hardest things for me because I was going to lose some of the best friends I had. I indeed felt as if I were a native Grenadian.

We took off from St. George's boat yard on one of the most popular boats known in Grenada. Almost as soon as the boat started to move, I started to vomit; and no matter the place in the ship I went to, I started to vomit protractively. I threw up so much that I had nothing else in my stomach for about ten hours that it took us to get to St. Vincent.

I got into St. Vincent very, very weak, and I was almost admitted for dehydration. Also, during this time, I had what I thought was a revelation. I began to feel that my grandmother and mother were by me and told me to have a change of my Nigerian roommate and also told me to get serious with my school work at this juncture. I was definitely weak, exhausted, and my mind wandered all over the place.

In St. Vincent, I found an apartment right in the middle of town in the business district of Kingstown. I became isolated unlike in Grenada where I was very popular. I took a low social profile here and began to learn more about medicine. I had a lot of rotations with British, American, and Irish doctors and teachers; and the most influential teacher and one who touched me and got my interest in medicine more stimulated was Dr. Cutler. Dr. Cutler was from Emory University in Atlanta, Georgia. He came to teach us and also to sharpen our patient presentation. During one of our town-hall-style lectures, I volunteered to present a case history; and after that, he was so pleased and came forward to me and told me that it was a thoroughly presented case and something his students in the United States could not do. If I needed any motivation to go through my clinical rotations, this was it.

I felt a wave of change and pride run through my artery and veins and said to myself that I was now on my way to becoming a real doctor. I wanted to be like Mbazoa who healed me but of the modern type. At this time I was so elated that I felt I would not feel my legs and my childhood life seemed to have come back to me. I could hear Mbazoa saying, "You can walk. Get up and walk," and I went back to my apartment after the class and prayed in all ways I could and thanked God/Allah for giving me an opportunity to undergo this experience.

After the clinical rotations in St. Vincent General Hospital, it was now time to either go to the United States or Britain or stay in the islands of Grenada or St. Vincent to complete the clinical rotations in medicine. This was also the time that one of the darkest aspects of the university came to light. The names of students and where they were to go for their clinical rotations were called out in the assembly hall. I was often one of few non-Caucasian-sounding names that were often called.

We the non-Caucasian students laughed about it, but it was not a laughing matter for those who had clinical rotations in the United States of America, Britain, or the islands. Majority of the non-Cascadian student were sent to Britain, and some were left on the island to complete their final year's work.

I was chosen to go to St. John's Episcopal Hospital in Jamaica, Queens, in the city of New York.

I was very delighted but still unhappy about what was happening to the other students who could not have the same experience. I later found out that one of the reasons I was chosen was because of Dr. Cutler's recommendation and also the fact that I did not owe the school any monies because my country, Ghana, had stuck to her commitment of getting me very well educated.

Medical Externship experience in American Hospitals.

I left St. Vincent for the United States on August 1982 through JFK Airport with three other African students. We arrived in New York not knowing a soul. A bus driver whom we later found out was a hustler decided to accommodate us, which ended up being a nightmare. We were threatened about payment of rent even though we paid him exorbitant rents three months ahead of schedule. On the second week after arrival in New York, we went to St John's Episcopal Hospital for an interview. From there I was told that my clinical rotations would be at Methodist Hospital in Brooklyn. At this time I had already rented a room. I decided to keep the rented room and to commute to Brooklyn via the A train of the New York City metro system to start my clinical rotations.

My first rotation was a twelve-week rotation in internal medicine with Dr. Adler who was a senior resident from St. George's University School of Medicine (the first class to graduate from St. George's University). This was the most motivating factor because I could finally see a product of medical education from my own university. I started the rotation very diligently and dedicated that I was going to shine during my first rotation in the United States. I worked hard, and even though I lived in Far Rockaway, I made sure I was never late to my early morning rounds. I was also the last student to leave the hospital when I was not on call. It was easy to identify me because I was the only student with Negroid features in my clinical rotation class.

At times at two o'clock in the morning, I could always be found in the subway on my way back to my residential area in Far Rockaway.

On one occasion, I went into a coach where there were four other gentlemen. All of a sudden, they began to discuss about their lives in prison. I immediately became afraid after I heard one of the passengers boasting how he had killed a person in a gang-related event. Whilst not making it obvious that I was hearing them, I had to find a way to prove that I was not scared or intimidated by these persons. At this time, I had an Afro-style hairdo; I quickly put my fingers between my long Afro hair and began messaging my hair and speaking in Mampruli (my African dialect) loudly. All of a sudden, I had a gaze from the four people, and they quickly got up and left the coach in which we were. My pulse increased at this time, and I was morbidly scared because I did not know where they had disappeared to. I stood up, looked around myself, and found no soul in the coach; so I walked the opposite direction the four had exited until I met a crowd of people in another coach whilst walking away from my initial coach. I could not count the number of times I prayed to God and all my ancestors, but I could feel a shadow guarding me away from where I sat before. When I got to the next coach where there were a lot of passengers, I felt more secure, but I still looked around to make sure my former four coach mates were not hanging around. Feeling more comfortable now and with the company of the crowd in this coach, I sat down and began to read Dr. Cutler's book on physical examination until I got to my destination about an hour later. I was still careful not to get out unto the wrong train station. Up-to-date, I cannot remember how I got back to my rented room.

In my internal medicine rotation, I was found a lot in the emergency room because on my call days, I had a lot of admissions. On one occasion, which I will never let out of memory, a young African American woman in her late twenties had presented with vomiting blood. Dr. Adler came to me and asked if I could take the admission since he thought she was going to be a difficult patient.

With my luck, I walked toward her to begin to take a history. I introduced myself and stretched my hands to greet her. She started shouting in a loud voice, "I do not want a nigger doctor. I do not want a black doctor." I got startled, and I stepped aback, hoping that reasonable minds would eventually prevail and convince her to be examined by me. As I stepped forward toward her, she started screaming again. This time Dr. Adler heard her and came over to speak to the woman. "I prefer a Jewish doctor like you than that nigger," she said in a melancholic voice. I was speechless but was well composed. I could not even think of words to respond to this ignorant person.

Dr. Adler took a step back and in a not-too-subtle manner told her that her insults were unwarranted in an emergency room setting. He came over to console me; at that time I was saying to myself she was losing an opportunity to be examined by one of the best student clinicians who was also in position to help her. I then stepped aside.

Dr. Adler told her that if she preferred another doctor, she had to wait until a non-black doctor could see her. After this incident, I went back and took over another African American patient without any hesitation. I did not think that lightning could strike at the same place twice in one day.

The patient started to talk about what she had overheard and how disgusting that was. I did not want to discuss an issue with her that she had no role to play. After seeing the patient, Dr. Adler came and felt that I was hurt, but I told him I was fine. "It is her loss not to have a good clinician take care of her and to help solve her problems," said Dr. Adler.

As if an angel were around me, I remembered my mother telling me that I should be patient in every aspect of my life because golden fruits are born from patience. I was still curious to find out why a black sister would think that I was incompetent solely because I was black like her. Could she be angry at all black mates, or was she unhappy about her own existence as a *human being*. I later found that this patient was one of the regular clinic patients. One day I was in the medical clinic when the same woman was sitting with her two children. One of the children could not walk and had some leg braces. As soon as I saw the child with the leg braces, almost immediately the memory of my childhood days overcame me. I was now very curious to find out why a black lady with a crippled child could on her own exhibit such hatred. Whilst I was waiting on a friend of mine to finish her clinic assignment, the woman came toward me to see if I could watch her child whilst she went to clean her younger child she was holding in her hand. She did not realize that I was the same black doctor she did not want to be examined by. She was now entrusting her child to be watched and played with by a man she had refused to be examined by. The kid she wanted me to watch was the crippled one in braces. When she came back, she thanked me. I was, however not, willing to let things go, so I asked her why she entrusted her crippled child to a person she did not know or was a complete stranger and not the only one in the clinic at that time.

She said, "Because you look very honest." I asked her if she knew to whom she was talking to. I recounted what happened in the emergency room to her and just wanted to know how she immediately equated the fact that I was black to incompetency. She said to me it's because all black lawyers and doctors in her community went to school because of affirmative action practiced by the schools and not because they were intelligent or competent. I could not believe what I was listening to an excuse like this for an equally stupid behavior. I explained to her that it does not mean when you go through on affirmative action program that the person is incompetent. She told me that view was held by her and many people in the Brooklyn community and the United States in general. Trying to convince this sister was a complete waste of my valuable time. She came through to me as if she was rather jealous of the African American professionals.

I asked her if everything was well with her, and she started expressing her frustrations as to how her two boyfriends had left her with two unhealthy children and how she resented black men in general. I began to see that this woman was frustrated and had wanted her turn to take her frustration on the wrong black man or professional she came by. I looked at my watch, and it was almost 6:30 p.m., and I excused myself and left.

I took up my bag after changing my clothing and went into the A train and went home. After talking to this woman, all of a sudden, it dawned on me that that woman could have been in the same position my mother was. Because of my experience of being disabled in childhood and because of the possible frustration my mother went through, I began to applaud my mother even though she had a very supportive husband who was loving and caring and who did not leave her alone to take care of me and my siblings. "Was my mother this frustrated and angry this way when I was disabled?" I asked myself. I sat in the A train and every thought came into my mind. I felt I was in my village, Bulbia. I actually felt sorry for the young lady, but I felt that some of her frustrations were brought on by herself. She was not only disrespectful to herself but did not care the number of people she hurt who crossed her path of hopelessness.

How could I tell anybody that this kind of bigotry or resentment was exhibited by a woman of my own race? It bothered me for a while, but I was too tired, and I quickly fell asleep when I got home and left all other thoughts to the next day.

The rest of my internal medicine rotation was uneventful. I worked hard and passed all my theory and clinicals in the twelve-week rotation; whilst I was in this rotation, I was thinking about the next rotation, which was to be a surgical twelve-week rotation. During our last week of the medicine rotation, every American citizen in our class had their rotations arranged. A lot of our schoolmates were from very wealthy homes, and a lot of them had medical doctors as parents. They had no problem setting up their rotations because of the connections they had professionally. I was informed that all the non-American citizen students were now going to England to complete their rotations in surgery, psychiatry, obstetrics and gynecology, and all the rest of the clinical rotations. I did not want to leave the United States this time to do any rotations in England.

One day about a week before the end of my internal medicine rotation, one of my professors came to the conference room where I was supposed to present two gastrointestinal bleeding cases. I was to present and discuss the cases from a medical and surgical point of view. Almost all the attending physicians attended this conference.

As if I knew my destiny was on this case, I prepared myself very well and presented both cases from a diagnostic, anatomical, and pathophysiological aspect of gastrointestinal bleeding. I presented the cases; and just as I was about to walk out of the conference room door, a voice called unto me, "Dr. Yamusah, come and speak to me.

I am going over to my office now, and I will like to have a word with you if you have any time to spare," said my surgical professor. I could not wait. I got to his office before he did and waited. I went into his office, and his secretary sent me in. He told me that the presentation and management of the cases was an impressive one and he wondered if I was going to complete my rotation in the Methodist Hospital in Brooklyn.

He congratulated me and told me how impressed he was with my presentation, and he said if I continued all my rotations like this, I was going to become a very good physician. After he spoke to me, I thanked him for his confidence. He assured me that if there was anything that he could do to help me in any way, I should call on him.

I quickly told him that my next rotation was in surgery since he had asked me the question. He asked me if I was going to do the rotation in the Methodist Hospital. I told him that there were not enough surgical slots, so I had to go somewhere else. He asked me if I was intending to go to England to complete my surgical rotation since he had heard that St. George's was sending some of her externs to England. He looked up to me and asked me if I really wanted to go to England. I hesitantly told him that I was not keen on going to England. He again looked up to me and said "You do not have to go to England to compete your medical studies. I will call my friend Dr. Ibrahim in Englewood Hospital in New Jersey and see if he can get you a space. I want you to get yourself up to Englewood Hospital by 7:00 a.m. to see Dr. Ibrahim tomorrow." I almost passed out when I heard these words. He asked me where I lived and asked me if I thought that would pose a problem.

In my mind I said if I can come from my village Bulbia, Ghana, one of the most remote villages in the world, there is no place that I cannot get to.

"Make sure you are there tomorrow," the professor reiterated. "He is reserving the only externship position for you in that hospital." I did not know how to thank him, and I started to express my emotions. At this point, I did not know if Englewood Hospital externship credits would be acceptable to St. George's University School of Medicine or not. I was going to a new place that later created a fertile ground for other students from my school.

For the rest of the day, I was in cloud nine. I was happy, but I had to prepare to go to Englewood. I got up and went and bought myself a new white coat and then left for my apartment. It was difficult for me to sleep as I thought I was going to oversleep and miss my appointments. I tossed all night long and finally woke up at three o' clock in the morning and was by the subways before five o' clock.

I took the A train to the Washington Heights train station and then took bus 166, which dropped me on Engle Street in Englewood, which was very adjacent to Englewood Hospital.

At the bus stop I met Tony Cefelli who had gone to school in Italy and was starting his rotations the same day. I went into the hospital and asked for Dr. I. Ibrahim's office and where I could find him. I was told that I was a little bit too early but that he would be in the office in a few minutes. At about 6.45 a.m. Dr. Ibrahim came into the surgical office. The secretary introduced us as I stood up in respect of Dr. Ibrahim, who was as elegant as I expected. "You come all the way from Far Rockaway, New York, and you are already here," he said. "Because of your promptness and your abilities described to me, consider yourself a member of the Englewood family." He asked me if I was ready to get started, and I assured him that I was enthusiastically ready.

He took me into his office and offered me coffee, and there began one of the most remarkable days of my life and the meeting of a great personality in vascular surgery and one of the most dignified human beings I have ever met. I registered the names of all patients examined and managed by me during my clinical rotation The reasoning behind this was because the St. George's University School of Medicine had not yet been informed of my acceptance to the Englewood Hospital teaching program. I did not know how the Dean of clinical studies would react to my being accepted to do my surgical rotation or externship in Englewood Hospital when I was slated to go to England like my other non-American citizen colleagues. What I did not know was that the school was delighted to have another program in the state of New Jersey they could affiliate with since my participation in this program could lay a foundation for others in the future. I took every aspect of this clinical program seriously.

After working with Drs. Abraham, Dardik, Kahn, and Sussman for some time, Dr. Ibrahim took me to the director of education's office and brought me a schedule of all the rotations I had left in my last year of my medical education. "You can show this document to your school," he said, "and if they have a problem with it, let them call me and discuss it with me." I was later to find out that he had already discussed with my Dean of clinical studies to inform him about this issue based on my experience in the school. As a precedent was set by any St. George's students, I decided to diligently keep all copies of my clinical rotations including case histories in case there were disputes with the school as to the authenticity of my externship. I continued to work hard, and on days I was on call, I slept in the on-call rooms designated for physicians and medical students on call. As if God and Allah were watching me, I was standing one day when a female employee who was later to be one of the most admired and trusted friends came to me and told me that I seemed and looked like a person who could keep his mouth shut. She offered me a small room in the nursing school and told me that it was unofficially mine to stay sleep and take my clinical rotation seriously because I did not have to commute from Englewood to Far Rockaway, New York, each day.

I was also given some food coupons to be used to purchase food from the hospital cafeteria.

My mother had advised me that the first thing to know or familiarize oneself wherever one got to a new environment was to get to know the coordinators or management of meals or food service. My mother's advice was probably due to the fact that because of cultural entities my brothers and myself were never taught how to cook or clean. Even when one tried to end the norm in out Kantonsi tribe one had to go through the humiliation of being called *poa nin dowa* (translated a man and woman).

Since my upbringing has been influenced by my parents' teaching and advice, after getting to a place in Englewood Hospital to lay my head and also now getting a source of getting food through the hospital cafeteria, I felt important steps had been set to set my mind free and happy. I made sure that nobody would ever know what was going on. I barely had enough money in my pocket at this time, and the above arrangement was not only being happy but grateful.

Essentially, I was flat broke, and it seemed that the Almighty and my ancestors had worked out one of their miracles again.

I did all the rest of my clinical externship program in Englewood Hospital, and I met a lot of students from other institutions; but in doing so, l made a lot at friends from all walks of life.

I was never born a sportsman; and because I was born crippled, I often made sure I did not participate in a sport, which was going to set me back to my old days. I often did not participate in any extracurricular activities except walking about three times a week. I liked walking into the wilderness after Tenafly and on Route 9 in Englewood Township. Walking was a very solemn period for me as I used those periods to examine and regenerate some new form of energy, relax, and enjoy myself.

I made every excuse not to attend parties in order to have enough time to study for my Examination Commission for Foreign Medical Graduates (ECFMG) and final written and oral examinations. In some parties, not only alcohol was being served openly but illicit drug inhalation was a known entity. I decided I did not want to get myself involved with peer groups and stuck to the idea of being left alone. Some people thought that I was too good for them. This farmer's son explained to them about my hesitance. I used these periods to study for my final examinations. I passed both of my school's final year examinations, which took place in St. Joseph's Hospital in Paterson, New Jersey, which was later to be the institution where I did my fellowship training in hematology and oncology.

My medical school graduation took place at the United Nations Headquarters in New York city. This was one of the loneliest events of my life even though I was accompanied by one of the best student friends. I often said that when I graduated from medical school, I was going to have my parents, grandmothers, grandfathers, and all my siblings to my graduation. I did not get this opportunity and luxury. I could not afford to pay for my parents' trip to the United States of America, and they could not afford to purchase air tickets to the United States of America. I surely wished my maternal grandmother would have been alive when I graduated. I wanted to hand deliver the diploma to her and walk with her to get the diploma from the school's chancellor. As reinstated earlier, my grandmother often thought that because I was constantly failing in school that was the reason I was not graduating from school to make her some money when I got a job after school. My grandmother had died in 1978, and I continued to "fail" because of my big head, which was empty and resulted in my numerous demotions. After the graduation, I went back to the hospital and rejoiced by myself. I prayed and thanked God for the opportunity of graduating from medical school.

Whilst I prayed, I remembered that in front of me was the issue of getting into a residency program. I had decided that I was much interested in internal medicine and was now seeking a residency position. The odds against me getting a residency position was the fact that I was a foreigner and added to it that I had graduated from a foreign medical school. This combination was to reduce my chance of getting a residency position in internal medicine, and it would be my next focus as time came along. I immediately wrote a letter home to inform my parents about my graduation. My dreams of one day becoming a medical doctor had started to bear fruit. I wanted to go home badly to hand my diploma to my mother who had believed in me and also to put my diploma on top of my grandmother's headstone and tell her that I finally achieved all that I wanted even though it took me so long.

A day after graduating from medical school, I went back to my room in the old nursing school dormitory in Englewood Hospital to rest. As I went in, I kept thinking of what I was going to do next in my life if I did not get a residency program. I had already decided that I wanted to be a specialist in internal medicine and not a primary care doctor.

However, I did not go through the national matching program that places recently graduated medical students into residency programs throughout the United States and Canada. I, however, never applied to be matched through this program for no specific reason.

As I walked past the entrance of the nurses' residences of Englewood Hospital after walking out of the new library one of the nurses called up to me that I was wanted in the medical staff office. I quickly ran back into the main hospital building and meandered my way back there in my infamous green surgical gowns and went inside the medical staff office. In the office before entering I saw the secretary of the medical staff who looked up to my face and handed me an envelope. I was very hesitant to open it and indeed had no single idea why I was called for. The secretary insisted that I open the envelope in her presence. I looked up to her and gently opened the letter and quickly noticed that it was an acceptance letter to start my residency in internal medicine on July 1, 1983. I was dumbfounded, but I was able to say thank you to the secretary; and as I left, something kept telling me that I deserved it. "You have worked so hard and sacrificed yourself to make your dreams come true," some strange voice kept talking to me. As I walked out of the medical education office, a cool gentle breeze blew and had a sign of relief. My fear of not getting a residency program without going through the national match program was settled. I took another step and then walked briefly to the cafeteria. As I went inside the cafeteria, a lot of my classmates, externs, and nurses came running to congratulate and celebrate the occasion with me. Somehow most of the residents in internal medicine had already known that I was going to be one of the new residents before I did. Their faces did not seem surprising to me, but they were happy for me. I felt bad for some of the externs who had rejection letters from the national match program on non-affiliated hospital programs. After eating with a group of my friends and other externs, I excused myself to say a prayer and to think about what was next. Some of my friends had organized a party for me at Club West in Englewood, but I could not go because some of the other externs although very happy for me looked dejected and worried. I did not want them to think that I was so selfish in celebrating in their midst of uncertainty.

As if the weight of the world had lifted off my shoulders, I wanted to cry, but I could not. I just wish my parents and siblings were around to appreciate this moment with me. I had finished all my notations and externships at this point, but I had not much to do.

After graduating from medical school in May 1983, I started volunteering to work with some of the residents in internal medicine program to get a step and see what I was going to get myself into. The third phase of Zara's Crippled Sons Life.

Residency Training in Internal Medicine in Englewood Hospital (NJ) and the onset of H.I.V. and AIDS Epidemic.

In June 1983 about two weeks, before my residency or internship was to start, the list of assignments were revealed for the new interns coming into the internal medicine program. I was to start off on the first of July 1983 rotating in the intensive care unit. Not only was I put in the Medical Intensive Care Unit (ICU) and Cardiac Care Unit (CCU), but I was also the first intern to take the first call of duty in the 1983 academic year.

I knew being selected to be in the ICU and CCU was an honor, and my fellow students and senior residents congratulated me on this issue. It was also a verification of my competency by the medical education staff that I could handle the chores. It was challenging, but I was incredibly prepared for the task ahead of me.

Since my days of remembering when I was crippled and could not walk and after I had traveled to many hospitals with my mother, I was finally going to get a chance to affect some other people's lives usefully. I believed I had a calling to be a medical doctor, and I said to myself and often remembered what my father would say, "If you are not enjoying what you are doing, don't only frustrate others but yourself too. People who go into medicine and were really naturally not meant to be one often are abusive not only to themselves but also to nurses, nurse aides, etc.; and they often become depressed with a sense of frustration.

If the happiness on this occasion was an indication of the type of love that I have for medicine, I was a very young man who was mentally ready for the hard work that lay ahead of me. I went back to the nursing school where there was a graveyard, and I took a cup of water with me and poured libation to my ancestors and deities through a window for all their spiritual power they and the Lord had given me, and I was mentally and physically ready to start my initial stages of my becoming a medical specialist.

Words cannot express the anticipation that abound me before the official beginning of the internal medicine program. I was, however, not too pleased because some of my class and school friends did not have residency programs and some could not pass their ECFMG exams. I had three days before starting my internship. I had enough time to sleep, and I slept so soundly I could not remember any event that happened that night except expressing my gratitude to everybody who supported my efforts to become a medical doctor.

On July 1, 1983, I was one of the first interns to show up the Englewood Hospital and ready to go to work. My first day's experience in the medical Intensive care Unit (MICU) and Cardiac Care Unit (CCU)started with a sixty-two-year-old white male who presented with signs and symptoms of an acute myocardial infarction. The patient was hemodynamically unstable with hypotension and bradycardia. As he became hypotensive, he also had electrocardiograph (EKG) changes commensurate with an acute inferior wall myocardial infarction with an acute right ventricular infarction. His blood pressure was low, and a lot of intravenous fluids had to be infused into him in order to keep his blood pressure stabilized. A call was placed tothe cardiologist, and it was decided that the patient was too unstable, and it was to transfer the patient to Montefiore Hospital in Bronx, New York, for cardiac catheterization and other cardiac management since Englewood Hospital did not have a catheterization laboratory at that time. On intravenous infusion the patient became more stable, but on the second day prior to transfer, he began to develop recurrent chest pains despite nipride and lidocaine drip, and the transfer was initiated.

Without thinking about it and since I was on call the night before, I hopped into the ambulance with the paramedical team and rode the ambulance to Montefiore Hospital. I was invited by the cardiac team to observe the procedure by the cardiac and open heart team.

After cardiac catheterization, it was determined that the patient did indeed have the right ventricular infarction with his inferior wall myocardial infarction; and when he was stable, he was transferred to the recovery room whilst I was still in the Montefiore Hospital.

After reviewing our management with the senior residents and cardiac fellows and was about to leave back to Englewood Hospital with the ambulance crew, a cardiac arrest was paged across the hospital. All of a sudden, a cold chill went throughout my body, and sweat poured out on me. After several minutes of resuscitating the patient, the admitting resident came to inform the Englewood Hospital team about their inability to successfully resuscitate our patient. He indicated that the patient had extended his prior myocardial infarction, and this culminated in cardiogenic shock.

Dr. G., the chief of internal medicine and senior cardiologist in Englewood Hospital, asked me how I was going back to Englewood, and I told him I was going back with the ambulance crew. He offered me a ride back to Englewood Hospital. Dr. G. looked back and told me how he was sorry I lost one of my first patients in ICU and encouraged me that if I continued to be diligent in my work as I have shown, I was going to have a very successful career in medicine and that it will go a long way to help build a good name for the residency program in our institution. I had no words to express since I was still thinking about my patient. I thanked him for his kind words and advice, and as we got to the hospital, I again thanked Dr Goldfisher for giving me a ride and the opportunity to participate in this wonderful experience. He shook my hand and said, "Young man keep the good work up," and left for the day.

The year of my Internship was when we began to see a lot of patients who came in with high temperatures and pneumonia. These cases were later known to be the onset of the Acquired Immunodeficiency Disease Syndrome (AIDS) cases. Most of our Hospital physicians did not even go into the rooms of suspected cases. The first cases of of HIV came from New York City because they did not want to be identified in the City. They came to Englewood Hospital to hide their identity in the setting of this mysterious disease that was killing a lot of patients. Until around 1984 when the French identified the HIV virus we classified this disease as Fever of Unknown Origin. In the hospital we were pronouncing dead about five patients a day with no knowledge as to how to treat these patients. Residents and students were the ones who were made to examine these patients and were in some cases the sole contact the HIV positive patient had contact with their health care team the whole time they were hospitalized. The outbreak of AIDS was similar to what is now going on with the current Ebola Crises. The initial cases seen were mainly white patients who had private attending doctors but because of the need for care and the unwillingness of the attending doctors to see their private patient, we were often allowed to follow these patients unlike other cases the private physicians would not put their patient under teaching if they had a choice. The majority of the teaching patients were often African American since there was a non-existent Hispanic population in Englewood at that time.

It was generally a very good experience throughout my residency period I learnt to deal with different doctors and their styles of applying the art of Medicine. One could easily identify those who were endowed with God's gift of applying the principles of medicine from those who went into medicine as a family business and those who just forced their way into the field of medicine. One also learnt and noticed the different communication skills that exemplified the different types of physicians we were exposed to. During the subsequent two years of being in residency, I kept a low profile and kept mainly to myself. I barely went out on social gatherings or parties. Working very hard was something I enjoyed. I could not be late for any event or not show up for any assignment because I was the only black in my class of Residents and the other black Resident was in the third year. I found myself being not only an ambassador of the Kantonsi tribe but a representative of the Negro race. I felt I succeeded as a representative even though some of my fellow Residents felt intimidated. I was doing something I always wanted to do with nothing handed to me on a silver platter.. I was often invited to go to parties, but I made every excuse to stay away. I had seen one of my former classmates being kicked out of his externship program which was a necessity for a medical student to graduate because of flirting with white girls, and the unequal treatment metted to the three black attending physicians who had privileges in Englewood Hospital and were employed or hired to stay quietly in the clinic..

In my mind, my aspirations in medicine had just began. I kept to myself even though I was called all kinds of names by my colleagues for not participating in activities they called fun. Some of the girls even went as far as spreading rumors that I was gay because of my refusal to accompany them whenever I was invited to parties or to go to the movies. Late in my second year of residency, I decided to apply to fellowship programs because of my desire to be a sub-specialist in Hematology and Oncology.. I applied to several places and got interviews in Downstate Medical Center, New York; Temple University in Philadelphia, Howard University in Washington DC; and St. Joseph's Hospital and Medical Center in Paterson in the state of New Jersey. After consultations with some of my professors and friends, I decided to do my sub-specialty training in St. Joseph's Hospital in Paterson, New Jersey.

What attracted me to St. Joseph's Hospital was my desire to study in an environment where a bone marrow transplantation program had just been initiated. I saw an opportunity to start a program to its fruition and to bring a very new program to the state of New Jersey. There was no Bone Marrow or Hematopoietic Stem Cell program available in the State of New Jersey and Bone Marrow Transplantation was in its infancy in the U. S. at that time..

After Dr. B., the program director, had interviewed me, i made my selection to do subspecialty training in Paterson, I was excited about having to get a new program of bone morrow transplant started, and also would be the only fellow since the senior fellow would be completing a two-year program in a few months.

I completed the residency program successfully, and the hospital had an end-of-residency party for all the third-year residents in the Englewood Hospital residency program. After this party I started moving to Paterson, New Jersey, in anticipation of beginning my fellowship and subspecialty training program. I also studied for my federal medical licensing board examination and passed it. xxxxxxxx

Sub-Specialist training in St. Joseph's Hospital and the establishment of the first Autologous and Allogeneic Bone Marrow Transplantation in New Jersey.

On July 1, 1986, I reported to St. Joseph's Hospital to start my fellowship. I took up residency in a hospital facility in a rented two-bedroom apartment. This residency was very convenient because it was very close to my place of work, and it gave me an opportunity to concentrate on my work.

Just before leaving Englewood Hospital, I was invited by one of the nursing assistants for a party. For some reason I made it. She had introduced me to her sister to whom I became friendly with, and I was sure her sister was going to be at the party. This beautiful girl did come to the party, but I found it hard to approach her. I however took notice and seemed for the first time that this girl had something special and turned on a key in my heart. I noticed her again on several times but again was too timid to approach her. I enjoyed the party and left, and this turned out to be the biggest gathering we had. We danced all night, and the next day I started moving to Paterson.

The program director was very helpful, and we worked very well with each other after I had started the program. In the hospital we could not be separated. I worked hard to initiate the autologous bone marrow transplantation, which had been started by the fellow before. It was in very rudimentary state. There were no protocols, and not much was retained in the registry of the hospital.

Gradually the hospital was able to get lamina flow rooms, which were later used for the first allogeneic bone marrow Transplant for a patient with acute pro-myelocytic leukemia, the first in the state of New Jersey.

I presented several reports of my transplanted patients to the New Jersey University of Medicine and Dentistry (UMDNJ) and to the Hematology and Oncology Society of New Jersey. I won first-place prize for fellowship research work on bone marrow transplantation held on a yearly event. It was presented by the UMDNJ Oncology Department in 1987.

At this point the autologous bone marrow transplantation in St. Joseph's Hospital was the first in the state of New Jersey. I was more than delighted to be a participant in a very virgin program. The transplant team group headed by Dr. B carried out about thirty-six autologous bone marrow transplantation and eventually channeled the program to a syngeneic and allogeneic bone morrow transplantation, which were all new programs in the state of New Jersey.

One of the exciting parts i played in the hospital was writing both clinical and nursing protocols for all the autologous bone marrow transplantations and for the first allogeneic bone marrow transplant in the state of New Jersey. The first allogeneic and syngeneic transplants were carried out in patients with acute pro-myelocytic leukemia and aplastic anemia in a twin respectively. All chemotherapy and supportive care programs were written out, and since this was the first allogeneic transplantation, i was very particular that nothing went wrong. I worked day and night on this new research project.. We also took a while to educate both the nursing staff and clinical staff that was involved in the transplantation program. The autologous bone marrow transplantation was carried out in Hodgkin's lymphoma, non-Hodgkin's lymphoma, acute lymphocytic leukemia (in adults), and breast cancer. We often would harvest the bone marrow in the operating room under general anesthesia. Bone marrow was then sieved to separate boney spicules and stored and when the patient had undergone intensification chemotherapy, the bone marrow of the patient was re-infused in the myelo-ablative or pancytopenic phase and monitored till the recovery of the bone marrow..

In some of the autologous transplantation, we attempted to introduce purging technics of the bone marrow in order to decrease the amount of diseased bone marrow that was to be re-infused into the patient through the Hickman catheter. I enjoyed all phases of bone marrow transplantation. Lymphocytes in the marrow were almost depleted from the bone marrow via purging, and this reduced the risk of allograft rejection and/or occurrence of interstitial lung disease, bronchiolitis obliterans organizing pneumonia (BOOP) as a complication of transplantation. With the first allogeneic transplantation, no purging technique was used even though we had a program in case it was needed in the future.

The first year of my fellowship was when I had my license to practice medicine in the state of New Jersey this enabled me to work in the emergency. My fellowship director who was also the chief of Internal Medicine had also recommended other fellows in Pulmonary and Cardiology also to moon light as Emergency Room Physicians. The Emergency Room work was done when we had completed our daily chores as Sub-speciality fellows in our own spare time. There was no interference and the hospital could rely on licensed fellows rather than Family Medicine Residents that they had come to rely on..

One of the main reasons why I wanted to work in the Emergency was that my boss and other physicians on staff were constantly expressing how badly run the emergency room was during our hematology rounds. When I inquired into who the chief of emergency services was, it was not surprising that the chief of emergency services was the only African American physician in the entire medical staff roster. I could deduct from some of my supervisors and some of the other Caucasian doctors comments that Emergency Room was being headed by an African American. The type of language that was used was very appalling and it came to me as if they were verbally chastising me personally. In fact, he was the only African American in the Department of Medicine, if not the entire hospital medical staff. He was also employed by the hospital. I was later to find out that there was no private African American attending in a hospital located in

Paterson where the population was predominantly African Americans and Hispanics, which was contrary to what was communicated to me to get me to commit to doing my fellowship in Paterson. Why is it that the second largest hospital system in the state of New Jersey had no private African Americans or Hispanics in private practice? I was later to find out why there were only one or two minority doctors on staff.

In the Emergency room, I got to know the relationship between the population of Paterson and the hospital as a health institution, the relationship between the city police and the transportation of prisoners to the hospital who were either injured by themselves or by others, and the sort of relationship that existed between St. Joseph's Hospital as a Catholic institution and the populous it collected millions of tax payers monies to take care of.. I also got to know the destitute and poor and often helped to feed the homeless breakfast whenever I could. I eventually got to know the routine of patients like Mrs. Lopez who took up to drinking alcohol after she lost her husband and her oldest son. There was a story behind every human being i met. People do not just get poor because they like poverty. Circumstances, usually psychological, have a severe impact on the vulnerable persons. The relationship between the two institutions often made reporting abuse cases impossible. When one was concerned how a prisoner got an injury while they were handcuffed, it was often deferred to abuse by another prisoner. Physicians like Dr. H who were vociferous and concerned about how the African American and Hispanic patients often come from the jail with suspicious wounds often did not have their contracts renewed. I also got to know the alcoholics and poor and often helped to feed the homeless breakfast whenever I was on call overnight. I eventually got to know the story behind every alcoholic or the homeless. Each patient had their unique history as to why certain things changed their lives. Mrs. Lopez very often would show up at a certain period of the day almost always drunk. She, however, unlike most Patersonian's could speak both Spanish and English rather fluently. I got to find out that she often went to the graveyard to visit her husband and son who had died before coming to the ER to get attention. She had to drink to get the strength and passion to visit the graveyard. There was a story behind every human being I met who came to the ER indigent and poor. In my case most likely because of my own experience with my senior brother, I respected and made friends with them. I was instrumental in improving the relationship between the populace and the hospital be it in the Oncology clinic, which I headed, or the Emergency room where majority of the population came to get care and some used the emergency room as a primary care facility.

In my third year as a fellow, I also rotated to St. Michael's Hospital under Dr. K who treated his fellows as if he was a slave driver. St. Michael's under Dr. K had no respect for his hematology and oncology fellows. I personally could not accept the way he disrespected his fellows even in front of medical students and residents because they were all immigrants.. One day after rounds i was very disappointed as to how he had treated his senior fellow (a third-year fellow) whom he had just embarrassed in front of everybody. I voiced my opinion to him after the rounds, but he was not used to listening to other people's opinion. After approaching him and he did not like it, we amicably agreed to allow me to go back to my institution. I went back to St. Joseph's Hospital and reported my experience. My director indicated that he was grateful to have me back to continue the bone marrow program, and since I was also a licensed physician unlike the fellows who were rotating from St. Michael's Hospital., I did not need any supervision to run the oncology clinic. He told me that he was not surprised that we did not get along but was grateful to have me back.

After two years of fellowship. I was the first fellow to start and successfully complete in St. Joseph's history the three year combined Hematology and Oncology program, I decided to spend the third year on research in solid tumor and autologous bone marrow transplantation. My goal was to set up and manage the first allogeneic bone marrow transplantation in the State of New Jersey. I got the opportunities to carry out a syngeneic transplant on a patient with aplastic anemia who had a completely matched related donor (twin). The patient after being treated with high-dose Cytoxan and the bone marrow infused went into remission and went back to Puerto Rico after the successful transplant.

I also at this time was making preparation for an allogeneic bone marrow transplant in a forty-six-year-old Hispanic male who had acute promyelocytic leukemia (APL) in first remission who was clinically unstable, did not go on a prolonged myeloablative phase, and was most likely to relapse. The first allogeneic transplantation involved organizing elements between the medical management team, the laminar flow room maintenance, and the education of the nursing staff and residents on this program as I had earlier alluded to..

At this time I had a few months left in my fellowship program, and I wanted the first allogeneic bane morrow transplantation in the state of New Jersey to be a success.

Since my fellowship was coming to an end, I had arranged with the hospital to have my visa changed to an H-1 visa, which I later found out was a bad idea, so that I could continue to work for the bone morrow transplantation after my fellowship. The president of the hospital signed my visa document after the erroneous advice from my attorney, Lawyer Essien who was a Ghanaian lawyer whom I thought was professional. Thinking that everything was well arranged and thinking that it was only going to take me the weekend to return from Barbados, in the Caribbean where I was scheduled to pick up my visa, i made arrangements for coverage in my absence.

It was a Friday, and I had informed the whole staff and my superiors and in my notes that I had to go to Barbados to pick up my extended visa that was signed by the president of the hospital. However, one episode seemed to change the relationship between me and my supervisor.

The president of the hospital and her clergy friends had left for México on vacation. On their return, the president had attained a laceration on her right hand and presented to the emergency room for help when I was the attending doctor on that day. When I saw the cut, even though I knew I could suture it, I decided to call for the plastic surgeon who was on call to take care of the President of the hospital instead of doing it myself. However, the plastic surgeon was taking too much time. The president who was a Catholic nun or sister decided to let me go ahead and suture her hand instead of waiting for the Plastic Surgeon on call.. I proceeded in suturing her hand, controlled the small amount of bleeding, and under sterile conditions bandaged the wound. She then received a tetanus toxoid vaccination and given wound care instructions and a prescription for antibiotics to make sure that the wound was not going to get infected. I then referred her to the surgeon on call for follow-up as was the emergency rooms policy. She was reluctant to follow up with the surgeon and actually requested me to remove her sutures when they were ready to come out. Unfortunately, the president sent for me to remind me of the suture removal when I was on my hematology and oncology rounds with my hematology Attending. The nurse who came to inform me called me and was not very discrete. She called out loudly for me from a distance and actually screamed, "Dr. Yamusah, Sister N wants you to come to her office." Immediately, my fellowship chief wanted to know how it was that I was being called by the president of the hospital. He immediately gave me a very nasty look, and he wanted to know the circumstance that led me to suture the hospital president's hand. It seemed to me at that time that I did not think much about it since it was on my free time when I was working in the emergency room that this suturing took place.

From this time I noticed a complete change in his attitude toward me. I started hearing comments like "The Yamusah boy thinks he is a big shot because he sutured the president's hand." I did all I could to defray my supervisor to forget this episode, but he never did. I did not know he had a daughter who was also finishing her fellowship in Montefiore Hospital whom he was grooming to run the bone marrow transplant program. He kept discouraging me from staying in the area to go into private practice which was not my intention. I wanted to continue to work up the transplant program for regional or world wide recognition.

It was a Friday, and after this incident, I decided to leave for Barbados, West Indies, to pick up my new visa. I wrote the name of the fellow who was to cover for me whilst I was away over the weekend and anticipated that I was going to be back to work on the Tuesday of the following week. I arrived in Barbados on Friday, and since the American Embassy was closed, I decided to travel to Grenada where a lot of friends and their families still lived. I also had lost my best friend in life, Boyo, to cancer, so I thought this was an opportune time to go to Grenada where I studied medicine to extend my condolences to his bereaved family and children.

I returned to Barbados the Monday and went to the embassy. I presented my documents that were given to me by my lawyer to the

consular clerk. She came back after a brief period of time on the
phone and demanded evidence of my medical training in the United
States. I pulled out all my residency certificates that I had attained
from Englewood Hospital and my first two-year certificate that I had
attained from St. Joseph's Hospital as well as my medical licenses
to practice medicine in the states of New Jersey and New York and
handed them over to her. She came back with a rather stern face,
looked at me straight in my face, and told me that she had just called
St. Joseph's Hospital in Paterson, New Jersey, and neither the chief of
the hospital nor the program director knew who I was. I immediately
thought that the counselor was joking or was going crazy. I also
thought that she was playing around with me.

At that time I could not believe what she told me, but later events
told what she had said was the truth. Another worker then asked me
after the stone-faced officer had left if I needed the telephone numbers
of the people they had just called. I therefore took the phone and
called my bosses' office, and the secretary whom I thought I knew very
well told me in an unfriendly tone that Dr. B was not available to me.
This secretary I had dealt with when I was in the hospital and often
professed her frustration of working in that environment to me seemed
as if she was hearing a voice from another planet. It was surprising
since all the secretaries in the hematology and oncology department
knew who I was. I then figured after I spoke to the secretary that if
these persons could not come to talk to me on the phone when they all
knew I was away, it was more than likely that they told the counselor
personnel that they did not know me. She took my documents and
told me to come back at the end of the week for her to find out what
was going on.

This time I decided to stay in Bridgetown, Barbados. I did all I
could to get in touch with the hospital and finally got in touch with
one of the Catholic Nuns who I had very good relationship with
because she was in charge of the emergency room service. Whenever
she needed somebody in the emergency room because another
physician failed to show up, she often called me to help fill the gap,
which I often did willingly in order to help run the emergency room
as smoothly as possible. I informed her what had happened and
everybody in the hematology/ oncology department including the

nurses and my chief knew about my absence. Shockingly on the phone she told me that my boss had told her that I did not inform him or anybody that I was leaving after setting up such an important research after I had worked on it for so long. I asked her how she was told, and now I began to realize that a game was beginning to be played on me. She was not as cheerful as she usually was and seemed to be in a hurry to end the conversation. Was this another distrusting element with a person or persons of the Catholic faith again? I asked myself because I knew they were all lying, and she in particular knew because I had also informed the emergency room of my pending short absence from work.

Realizing that some respected religious persons had begun to fail me again, I did not lose my composure once I realized the game that was attempted on me. She was very resistant in some of the things she said since she did not want to implicate herself in any way.

On the Friday I returned, and the counselor told me that she could not still get a person to tell them if I had ever worked there or not. She wanted to verify my fellowship position.

I thanked her and quickly decided I was going to go back to St. George's, Grenada, where I had some good friends who were not like the ones who had just let me down. I called St. Joseph's Hospital and told some of my friends who all knew all my plans what had happened. The president of the hospital even denied that she had signed for the extension of my visa, and my director did not still acknowledge that he ever knew who I was or ever saw me.

What surprised me more was that I was not perturbed or annoyed with these reactions. I was used to being disappointed, but to be disappointed by my chief and the president of St. Joseph's Hospital who was also a nun was an understatement. It quickly brought back the negative experiences I had when I was an exchange student in Bloomer, Wisconsin, and a priest let me stop serving mass because I was making him lose their congregation because a black boy was serving mass. Even though he did not tell me to quit, I put things together and stopped going to church because I was not only concerned that my serving mass was the problem but my presence in the congregation could result in an unwarranted consequence and further prevent his church's economic success because of this black boy's desire to serve his Lord in the same building we all professed to love people. I decided that I was not going to sit down and waste my time calling and begging people to tell me the truth. The hospital's representative knew what it was all about. I had been told by the same hospital authorities how excellent a physician I was, and that is all that mattered to me. They also knew that I was a dedicated physician who also loved his profession. This attitude of my doing the best to be recognized was not for a minority doctor. As a minority doctor, you were not to love medicine but take the profession as only a source of making money. There is also an understanding that for an African American doctor to be recognized, he had to be more than twenty times better than one's competition to even get a mentioning of one's name. These were the odds I faced with other blacks in the profession. I thought of all the hard work I had put into starting a bone marrow transplant program that was less than a year old and the time I spent in promoting; however, I was not scared or frightened as to the success or failure of my future, but I was rather strengthened to practice medicine the best way I could. "What happened to Zara's crippled child?" I asked. I had resolved that humans could fail me, but God and my ancestors have never forsaken me. I also decided not to contact my parents because they would be worried. I was now a grown man and the medical subspecialist I always wanted to be and no longer just Zara's crippled son. In a gesture of defiance, I looked up to the sky, gave my grandmother Amina a fist and a hit to my left chest, and felt ready for any challenge ahead of me.

After a week in Barbados, I went back to Grenada where I rented an apartment in one of my friend's cousins' apartment complex. After a week I decided to seek employment and to put my expertise as an internal medicine specialist and a subspecialist in hematology and oncology to use and to help the people of Grenada where I had attained my basic medical education whilst I was waiting for my visa to be approved.

Working as a Physician Specialist and Consultant in Grenada and my first experience with a Political Medical Directive and Mr. Kwame Toure (Mr. Stokely CarMichael).

I t was in April 1989, and I had a month left to complete my third-year fellowship in hematology and oncology. I was the first fellow to start the three-year program in St. Joseph's Hospital. I was also one of the few fellows who were paid for the three years except from March to June 1989. Most of the fellows in cardiology, pulmonology, and gastroenterology were often paid for the first year; and for the subsequent years they were told that the hospital had no funds for them to continue their programs. Most of them had to self-sponsor their way to complete their fellowship program. I was often envied by my colleagues, but none of them worked as hard as I did or brought up new and innovative programmes to the hospital as I did. In fact, medical residents from India and some Arab countries were being sponsored by their own governments and were not paid by the hospital. Some of my fellow fellows who completed the first-year programs had no choice but to sponsor themselves by working either as house officers or emergency room doctors in order to support themselves whilst they tried to complete their second-year programme. Again I was one of the lucky and hardworking fellows who was paid for the whole three-year program, and I worked very hard and brought new programs to the hospital. My fellowship achievements were often documented in the hospital's *Century* magazine from 1986 to 1989 along with my boss Dr. B. Most of the pictures taken for this magazine at this time was done by Mr. MK, who later became a Paterson City councilman and the ombudsman of the hospital.

With this experience, I was hired as a physician specialist in internal medicine, hematology, and oncology; and I worked hard to strengthen the programs in the St. George's General Hospital, which was a very familiar place to me where I did some of best externship programs as a student.. There were many hematology cases in the St. George's General Hospital. A week after I got there, i diagnosed a case of acute lymphocytic leukemia and several cases of HTLV-1 associated lymphoblastic lymphoma, which my best friend Boyo Thomas had died from and which is actually a sexually transmitted retroviral disease. I was pretty set and did not have much of a transition since i was already familiar with the surroundings and had also already worked with some of the best-trained, capable, and hardworking nurses in the world. There was no comprehensive blood banking program, and there was hardly any chemotherapy and other antineoplastic agents. I made use of what was available and made people better. I felt at home in St. George. My apartment in Blue Danube, a suburb of St. Georges was very comfortable. I lived on the first floor of my friend Boyo's cousin's house. Mr. and Mrs. Steward treated me as if I was a family member and introduced me to the various political and economic powers in the island of Grenada. Mrs. Steward made my stay in St. George's very comfortable.. Activities in the hospital was too busy and I barely had any down time to be lonely except for my fiancée that was left in the U. S. People personally came and thanked me for the good work I was doing on the island. Many people who could not afford to pay me in their expression of their appreciation brought me eggs, yams, and breadfruit; as such I never had to buy food whilst in Grenada. People were genuine and very appreciative of whatever was done for them, and it made the practice of medicine enjoyable and delightful. Ironically, after one month in the island, l was approached by the American Peace Corps Organization in Grenada to be their physician in Grenada. Here I was refused a visa extension by the American embassy, but I was thought good enough to take care of Americans under the same government's umbrella. I chuckled about it and took the responsibility for their care as well as the care of American or Canadian tourist who came to Grenada General Hospital and I got paid handsomely for my work.

One of the experiences that made me to double my efforts to leave Grenada involved political medicine, which up to that time I had not experienced.

One evening, whilst carrying out my duties as the Medical Consultant on call, the Sister called me to evaluate a gentleman who was in his sixties and had come from Africa to celebrate an anniversary of the former president of Grenada, Maurice Bishop's assassination. Prime Minister Maurice Bishop was assassinated during the U.S. inspired invasion of the Island of Grenada in the nineteen eighties, to protect American medical students in St. Georges University at the time. The gentleman drapped in an entire African attire gave his name as Mr. Kwame Toure. I walked into the ward accompanied by my students, two Residents and nurses, to see this patient who at this point was shaking like a leaf with a temperature of 105 degrees Fahrenheit on his bed and listless.

In my mind the name sounded very familiar but how could the man who was associated with name be doing in Grenada?, I asked myself. I knew the first president of Ghana was Dr. Kwame Nkrumah who had led my dear country Ghana to its independence from colonial British rule in 1957, and the president of Guinea in West Africa at that time was Mr. Sekou Toure. As a kid, I remembered in Ghana that Ghana and Guinea had a liaison and special diplomatic relationship. This man looked very familiar to me. I had seen his face on television, before but I could not in my mind remember who he was. Mr. Kwame Toure seemed to have been derived from the first and last name of two of the greatest presidents and leaders of Africa.

After going through my memory box and could not still recollect where I had seen Mr. Kwame Toure, I remained very professional in the private ward of St. George's General Hospital. I diagnosed him clinically to be suffering from malaria, and after some blood was drawn from him and intravenous fluids was initiated, I then left the ward with my residents to look at the thick peripheral smear in order to confirm our suspicion of malaria as a cause of Mr. Kwame Toure's symptoms.

After reviewing the peripheral smear and the laboratory work, I was more than convinced that Mr. Kwame Toure had malaria.

I started him on chloroquine and was monitoring the patient who at this time had developed some more rigors and cold sweats.

Even on his hospital bed, he seemed to have attracted a lot of people. There were people in the hallways and in the common areas of the private ward in the Grenada General Hospital. This by itself told me that Mr. Kwame Toure had to be somebody special. I would take a glance at him and try to recollect his face, but I was consumed in his management that I could not recollect him no matter how hard I tried.

The next day I got a directive from the Prime Minister of Grenada's office through the chief medical officer who was Dr. Y to discharge this very ill man because apparently Mr. Kwame Toure had left the wards in the late hours of the night to attend a political rally. I could not confirm this with the hospital nurses or security guards. The nursing staff had no indication that he had gone to a political rally to honor the late Mr. Maurice Bishop, the ex-President of Grenada who was brutally murdered during Mr. Reagan's induced invasion of the island of Grenada. The nursing staff had no indication that he had gone to the rally as reported by the Prime Minister, and to me a patient with a blood pressure of 85 systolic could not have lasted there for the length of time he was purported to have been out of the ward as alleged by the Prime Minister's office. I then asked the security guards why the Prime Minister of Grenada's office would be so interested in Mr. Kwame Toure's whereabouts. It was then and only then that it occurred to me that I was dealing with one of the greatest African American civil rights architects who was previously called Mr. Stokely Carmichael, the president of the Student Non-Violent Coordinating Committee (SNCC) of the civil rights era. I had read and heard of Mr. Stokley Carmichael and the important role he played and the sacrifices he made in order to liberate the Negro and the disenfranchised in the United States of America. I also know that he had moved back to Africa, so I was not surprised that he had taken the name Kwame Toure in honor of the two former presidents of Ghana and Guinea. I also knew he was born in Trinidad and a committed freedom fighter who studied Garveyism and the African in diaspora and actually practiced it by going back to Africa and marrying a beautiful African musician by the name of Ms. Miriam Makeba. I enquired from some of the people who were around him and was finally told the truth. I knew he had repatriated to Guinea and was living there. Even in my hour of enthusiasm of meeting such a great and honorable man, I still remained professional and continued to monitor his health until his status began to improve. He, however, was still on IV fluids because his blood pressure was still low when I was ordered to discharge him. I sat down with the representatives of the Ministry of Health and the nurse in charge of the ward(Sister) to express to them how unstable the patient was. The Sister seemed not to understand our responsiblilty as medical personnel and was very concerned that I was not discharging the patient after a Prime Minister's directive. I expressed to the administration of the Hospital my responsibility as a Medical Consultant taking care of a politically charged case, in the meantime using his low bliood pressure as a parameter of instability.. It was also expressed to them that i could not succumb to political pressure to discharge Mr. Kwame Toure who was still medically unstable and was still symptomatic from his malaria. "How can we discharge this patient who can barely walk or stand up?" I asked the sister. "Clinically this patient is too sick with malaria to be discharged," I said to myself. I prayed for God to give me the strength and power to get Mr. Kwame Toure better. I therefore agreed to disagree with the order to discharge him from the hospital. I considered the order a political order and not a clinical one, and it was the first time as a medical practitioner that I was going through this.

At about 8:00 a.m. the following day I was met in my office by a different sister (nursing supervisor) on call who came to remind me that the second presidential order had been sent for me to discharge Mr. Kwame Toure. I told the nursing supervisor that under international law and the Hippocratic oath that I had sworn during my graduation from medical school I could not be forced into discharging a hemodynamically unstable patient on political grounds.

I told the nursing supervisor that if the chief medical officer, Dr. Y, wrote the discharge order, then he could be discharged; but I was not in any position going to comply to a politically motivated order. The next morning, when I came to do my rounds, the patient Mr. Kwame Toure had been discharged in the darkness of the night by the chief medical officer with "stable vital signs," information that was definitely erroneous. I later found out that because Mr. Kwame Toure had come to the island of Grenada to celebrate the ex-President of Grenada, Mr. Maurice Bishop's assassination. He was not welcomed by the ruling party of Grenada because he was invited to the Island by the Opposition party,

I again objected to the decision and I made it clear to Dr. Y as the chief internal medicine consultant on the case. I expressed to the chief medical officer how upset I was over the interference of political opinions over the practice of medicine.

From this day onward, I never felt comfortable or safe in Grenada anymore. At one point I was more than prepared to make a long commitment to work in Grenada even though I was not on the same pay scale as a white expatriate without the qualifications I had. I also started getting strange visitors in Blue Danube, and my Landlord advised me not to accept rides from people not known to me after this incident. It was not unusual for me to be walking for a car to stop to offer me a ride. I refused several such rides often before because I had lived up Blue Danube, which was a hill, and by walkingking I had a lot of exercise and lost a good amount of weight that I had gained in the U.S. due to lack of exercise.. I actually enjoyed walking up the hill because I did not have enough free time to exercise. After this political incident, I refrained from getting car rides as adviced; Instead of walking home, I was often driven home by the hospital ambulance crew if and when it was late. I never felt safe in Grenada anymore and stepped up efforts to get back to the United States.

There were several interesting cases that I handled even though there were very meager resources in the hospital. I tried to raise up an issue to get the airlines that flew in and out of Grenada to contribute to an infrastructural buildup of emergency medical resources and apparatus in St. George's General Hospital.. The General Hospital, which was also the main hospital in the island, then had only one ambulance available in case there were emergencies on the island. On the other hand, this ambulance was also responsible for transporting nurses, doctors, and other hospital staff to and from their homes. When there was a true emergency, Grenadians were often found carrying injured persons by private vehicles, public buses, or sometimes with their bare hands running with the injured to the casualty (emergency) room. It was proposed that by putting this emergency infrastructure on board, it could help the airlines if and whenever there were emergencies involving the airlines or if airline workers were ill and needed emergency help on the island.

I came up with a plan to describe the potential crises that could occur if by chance an air disaster occurred and we had surviving casualties. We had no respirators, defibrillators, or ambulances to convey the sick and severely injured to the hospital from the two airports in the country.

After discussing this issue with the chief medical officer, he did not discourage me, but he added that this request would involve a long application request and would require approval from the Minister of health and the Prime Minister even if I was able to get private funding for the project through th airlines.. Knowing that I had already been involved with an ostentatious issue involving Mr. Kwame Toure, I did not think it wise to push an issue that could alienate me further, so the proposal was dropped. It is an issue that still worries me up-to-date because numerous flights go to Grenada, which has a very big and elegant medical school but the infrastructure of the medical center is still rudimentary at best. Any unforeseen disaster will remain so since there are no respirators or other emergency necessities that would be warranted in a dear emergency. When I think of Ghana, xx I find out that Grenada handles its medical system as other third world countries. If the prime minister or ministers are ill, they will prefer to go to other countries and become "charity care" patients in those countries rather than use their foreign aid or national income to improve their health care system. Most of the time, when they go to the United States, England, or France, they end up at the mercy of the host government or they never return to their country alive due to subpar treatment meted to them. On the other hand, one never hears of a donor nation building a modern hospital with all its equipment for an emerging nation but will give the aid to buy the most modern and sophisticated weapons to use on their own population whom when injured cannot find a decent hospital to send them to. The donor nations will rather have sophisticated health ships docked along the ocean so that the country will use the IMF or World Bank loans to pay for the health care facilities on the same ships. No wonder these countries continue to stay poor as more and more loans in the form of foreign aid continue to be poured into the corrupt politicians' pockets. The current Ebola crises shows us how vulnerable African countries are and are at a greater risk of neo-colnialism. The so called developed will compete to send soldiers and weapons in Ebola infected counties instead of empowering the local people with medical equipment that suit the climatic conditions in these countries. The rich nations encourage virology research in institutions such as run by schools such as Tulane University. When unforeseen mutations occur in these laboratories then the West African is blamed for eating bats and Chimpanzies when these practices have been in existence for thousands and thousands of years, Africa is blamed for HIV and Ebola when even the first cases of Ebola Rhesus did not even occur in Africa. Ebola rhesus was firsr identified in the Virginias when chimpanzee meat was brought into this country from the Phillipines. Africa is always blamed for the bad and the worst but the world does not even know the hunt for fine minerals for cell phones that improvises the African environment results in the world getting minerals etc at the expense of the Africans. Our politicians in their desire to please the world, often falls for every gimmick the United Nations puts forward with no thought given as to the implications of those polices to the African. The politicians are like prostitutes who only lie in bed, have sex they hardly desire or need but yet have one hand in the pocket to be paid after they have participated an act that should be so special between lovers.

The medical school in some way was not used by the political establishment to help structure the hospital and modernize some of the programs. A lot of money changed hands in order to make things politically suitable for the institutions, but none was used to make the health care system attractive enough for the basic Grenadians. There were a lot of foundations who sent congenitally deformed kids and other deformed children to the United States for care. The health care infrastructure was left undisturbed. Hospitals were built for the islands, which became giant infrastructures with nobody using them as seen in countries such as Antigua.. Isn't it the same story for most of the developing countries? Politicians are often helped to set out of their countries and go to the West or East only to stand in the charity care corridors. If they had used the monies given for aid to build modern medical institutions and encouraged the exchange of talent with the African diaspora, they would have had enough medical doctors who are competent enough to run those institutions. It is often embarrassing to see a whole Minister of State in another country or a member of parliament indicating to the populous they represent that they are going for care abroad—which, by the way, is a status symbol—only to end up in charity care rooms of hospitals or hospital clinics with no quality care and often return to their country in well-designed coffins after the inevitable has occurred. These African leaders don't even see that their own Africans in the diaspora in England the U.S. do not even get the best of care in a system ladened with prejudice. They rape the countries they represent and spend thousands to millions of dollars only to be sent back to Africa in decorated coffins succumbing to the same prejudice that has existed in the health care systems for decades.

I also started teaching the nursing students biochemistry and hematology and basic internal medicine. Grenadian Nurses are some of the most dedicated nurses I have ever worked with even though they have very little in terms of medical equipment. Their dedication to the profession is unquestionable. Most of them have to forego personal relationships in fear of getting pregnant and losing their ability to study nursing. Whether this takes a toll on some of the nurses or not is not known and to the best of my knowledge has not been of any of the concerns of the ministry of health when I worked there. The nurses in Grenada were also very well trained and could participate in procedures that the doctors who were doing their housemanship (internship) could not do. Their dedication to the island was very admirable even though they worked for meager salaries.

I worked hard to get a continuing medical education program especially for the general practitioners who were in the countryside and also in the sister islands of Carriacou and Petite Martinique. The continuing medical education (CME) program started very well with huge attendances. Eventually the program succumbed to a division between the Western-educated doctors and those who were trained in Cuba and the Eastern countries. This division is also in the political line, and one could not be neutral. You had to declare which side you belonged, or one was chosen for you, and criticism started in all ways. It divided the scope of medicine on the island and sometimes affected the health of the same people whose only responsibility was asking for help.

As an African, it was very exciting for me in Grenada because as a student I got to know and love Grenada very much because of my involvement in community affairs in almost all parts of the island. So as a physician, it was much easier for me to assimilate. A lot of people just called me the "African doctor"; and people came from all over Grenada, Carriaccou, and Petite Martinique. I also went to Carriaccou to do physicals on employees of Blue Danube Bakery that were located there on behalf of my friend and owner Mr. and Mrs. Stewart.

After the episode of Mr. Kwame Toure (Stokely Carmichael) in the hospital, some important air and zeal was pulled out of me, and I was never comfortable in Grenada, so I started working diligently to go back to the United States. I did not want to go back to my country without completing my bone marrow transplantation thesis that I was in the middle of completing. I had the end of May 1989 to complete my fellowship program in bone marrow transplantation when this ill-fated trip took place, but I had no regrets because I learnt a lot about the people I worked with and even learnt much more about myself and my ability to adopt to circumstances and make the best of them. As a physician, I found out that I could survive anywhere in the world.

One evening, whilst I was sitting, my girlfriend, who was left behind in the U. S. was brought to me from the airport to my apartment in Blue Danube, St. George's. It was a really nice thing for her to come to visit me and her presence was very much appreciated. I really appreciated her and admired the courage it took for her to come to an unknown country to look for her boyfriend. In some conservations with Mrs. Steward, I had indicated that if my girlfriend came to Grenada to look for me when I did not ask her to then, she cared and her hand will be sought for marriage When she came, she was confronted with this request she accepted to my surprise and agilation.. The ensuing events will be pursued in another section. After my girlfriend and my future wife left Grenada after her visit, more effort to return to the United States was made by me..

At this time a request was made for me to be the physician specialist for the Peace Corps group in Grenada. It was ironic that the same person who was denied a visa to return to the U.S. was now being asked to be responsible for it's citizens in Grenada. I was actually becoming more comfortable and would have stayed in Grenada if it's not because of my future wife and my research thesis, which was completed in Grenada before I got back to the United States of America.

Return to U.S from Grenada and the Completion of my fellowship in Hematology and Oncology.

I left Grenada in late November for Canada. I was on vacation from my consultancy position at that time. I eventually went back to the United States of America via Greyhound bus from Toronto. I showed all my documents at the border and had no problem getting a visa. So via Greyhound I left Toronto for New York City. All this time not a soul or my wife was informed of my return to the U.S... I went home to my condominium in Yonkers, New York, and then called my wife to inform her of my return to the United States. She did not believe me, and so the whole family was very surprised when I drove to her house in the Bronx. In one dream, I had dreamt that my wife was pregnant, but I had not popped the question; but when I reached her mother's house, she told me to my delight and adulation. I could not believe that she was pregnant of our first child. I was proud and very happy about becoming a father and I was mentally ready for the challenge..

Despite the fact that I was very tired, I did not want to sleep in my mother- and father-in-law's house in the Bronx, New York. I took off with my wife back to my condominium in Yonkers. It was the biggest surprise and gift she told me. I made sure I did not inform her that

I was on my way back from my ill-fated journey but I was delighted and grateful to God for giving me the opportunity to return without any problems and to surprise the institutions and my colleagues who were intrigued about my absence and who actually wished my disappearance from the face of the earth. I strongly believed and still believe it up-to-date.

The Monday after I came back to the United States of America, I did not inform St. Joseph's Hospital in Paterson that I had returned. After speaking with my wife, I left for St Joseph's Hospital and went straight to the office of the Chief of Hematology, internal medicine, and oncology's office. He was not in the office at the time. I could see the unbelievable staring and surprise bestowed on me from the secretaries who had spoken to me when I was in Barbados. They were subdued and shocked. The secretary informed me of the absence of Dr. B in the office and wanted me to return later to speak to him My request to sit down and wait for Dr. B was granted so I sat down and waited until he came from whichever place he was. They offered me a seat in the office, and then I could hear them whispering, "How did he get back into this country?"

I did not dignify them but held tightly to the Bone Marrow Transplant thesis I had written and completed for my research in the third and final year of my three year Fellowship in Hematology and Oncology.. The topic was "Bone Marrow Transplantation—a New Therapy for Neoplasia in the State of New Jersey." The secretary came back and told me that my fellowship certificate was being held up because I had not presented my research thesis. I could see the surprise on every eye of the secretaries who looked as if I had resurrected from the dead.

I was very respectful to them and did not want to stoop low to them as they did to me. They still looked very perplexed as if I had first dropped through the roof of the office or from Mars..

When my fellowship chief came into the office, he could not say a word for almost ten minutes, and I could see the perplexed state he was in. I opened up apologizing for my absence from the hospital for the month that was left for me to complete my fellowship.

What had transpired was not discussed because his and his secretary's reaction was enough to tell me that they had denied to the

America embassy in Barbados personnel that they did not know me. It seemed I did not exist in this world. I did not show any emotions, hostility, or agitation to my boss because of the respect I had for him. There is a proverb in my Kantonsi language that if you follow a mad man and act like one, then you will eventually become one. I would not follow the path of hatred. I was now qualified both academically and morally to stoop that low.

I discussed where I was with regard to my research project before this debacle in my life started. Interestingly enough, he did not inform me as to how the first allogeneic bone marrow transplant had gone after I had researched and written all the protocols and made the preparation toward its initiation.

He instead instructed me to outline the project on all the autologous bone marrow transplants and the preparative regimen of the allogeneic bone morrow transplantation and complete my thesis for him. I had the thesis with me, but a copy was not yet made for my records. I was not going hand in my thesis without getting my third year Diploma. I went out, made a copy and returned. Dr. Rubin gave me my Diploma and I thanked him for giving me an opportunity to do my Hematology and Oncology Fellowship with him. We shook hands and I left his office concluding my Sub-speciality training in three years, the first Hematology and Oncology Fellow in St.. Joseph's history to do so.

What I did not know was that this was to begin a more interesting relationship between me and my fellowship boss, whom I so much admired and worked hard for.

I also took back my job as a part-time emergency room physician, but this time the nun in charge was not going to get me into volunteering for more hours for the emergency room calls and calling me at odd times to fill spaces for other physicians who did not show up at their scheduled times or did not show up at all. Zara's crippled son was now wiser and knew more about human behavior. One is only wanted or reverred when one is in sight. When one is out of site no one remembers the good the person did and one can become a focus of lies and innuendoes.

In the emergency room I started hearing about the lies that was perpetuated on me while I was in Grenada. I did not dignify them, but the relationship with some of the Nuns and hierarchy of the hospital was never the same. I even gave away a green shirt Sister E had given me when I sutured her hand to charity. I had cherished it so much that I hung it in a separate closet; but because of the image it stood for and the disappointment in a human being especially a clergy, it was too much for me to let it remain hanging in my closet. It reminded me of not only being prevented to serve mass in a Catholic institution by a Catholic priest in Bloomer Wisconsin but also of the small church in the slave dungeons in the Cape Coast and Elmina Castles in Ghana where slaves were raped and brutalized by the same people who controlled the church.

The rumors and lies were flying from place to place, but I did not dignify them because they were being made to cover up the distrust they had created in the view of all the workers who saw through the lies. I decided after a while not to work for St. Joseph's Hospital's Emergency Room anymore especially when i could not even get an application for privileges in Hematology and Oncology. I left everything to the Almighty, my ancestors, and deities to handle all the non-human attributes of this chapter of my life.

A lot of the same people who were involved in creating lies or spreading rumors encouraged me to be angry and be disrespectful to the hospital hierarchy, but as my mother always told me, when you are angry, you lose your protective guard and your enemies or so called friends can then use that opportunity to further destroy one's good reputation. I had worked hard to build up a reputation in the Paterson community by taking care of patients in the AIDS clinic when no other Fellow would for fearing of contracting the virus. My philosophy is that if I should die or contract a disease entity because I was doing my job as a physician then I have fulfilled God's wish. I will never not take care of a patient because I was afraid to die. People like Dr. Salia of Sierra Leone should be recognized for his non selfish devotion to the people of Sierra Leone for dying from the Ebola virus whilst he was working . However the world should be ashamed that a person who contracted a disease from his work could not get help at the appropriate time because his family had to promise to pay back all transportation money before he could be transported to a Nebraska hospital to meet the inevitable was not only appalling but disgraceful.

The Caucasian doctors in Liberia were transported back to the U.S through Government intervention. When it came to helping a black doctor on similar circumstances the younger doctors care was delayed because of certain demands that were made of the already stressed family that resulted in the delay in transportation that culminated in the death of a doctor who was younger that the previous cases. Who says race does not matter in America in an era we claim to have our first Black American President.. One never head about demands made to all the Caucasian patients who were flown home at appropriate times and survived the brunt of Ebola.

As I always do, I resorted to my childhood and Zara's crippled son youth when my sisters, cousins, brothers, and so-called friends would often step on me and run because they knew I could not catch up with them. My mother always cooled me down and told me that one day they will answer to their wickedness. I was slowly beginning to come back in to American life after a six-month absence. A program was available in Harlem Hospital in conjunction with Columbia University Hospital in Manhattan, New York. It was an HIV research program that was under the auspices of the National Institute of Health in collaboration with Columbia University in Harlem Hospital..

I applied for this position because of my experience in writing research protocols and my experience in working in the HIV clinic at St. Joseph's Hospital when no other doctors would touch AIDS patients. This protocol-laden project involved a participation in writing protocols for the HIV research studies I was to be under the supervision of the chief of infectious disease, Dr. Elsadie in Harlem Hospital, as well as other physicians. I took the job because it was closer to Yonkers and also because it was on AIDS, where I had a lot of experiences having worked in the HIV clinic with Dr. R for three years. My wife at this time was pregnant, and I wanted to be close enough to home in case she ever needed me urgently.

I started working in Harlem Hospital, New York, but there was not much to do. On the days we had the HIV clinic, I felt my talent was not used. Majority of the time it seemed fruitless, and i hated walking around or sitting in the library all day doing nothing because the project documents had not yet arrived from Washington. I was particularly concerned about the cost to the system intubating every

Tom, Dick, and Harry who came through the AIDS department because we did not have a family liaison unit that could inform families of the grave news of their loved ones before putting them on respirators to lie there suffering sometimes for several months.

Also in Harlem Hospital, even though, I was a hematologist and oncologist, some of the students who were white and the white members of our team were respected, but often the minorities in the group had a lot of resentment from the minority nurses we came in contact with and were barely assisted when we asked for help..

It was difficult to get help since almost everything you asked a nurse or nursing assistant was not in their contract even when they were sitting doing nothing and painting their nails. I spent more time in the library on days I was not assigned to the HIV clinic or having rounds with the infection disease team. I did not feel I was enjoying the job. Realizing that my full talent was not used and the environment was not challenging a decision was made to re-focus my mind on what was my preference and leave Harlem Hospital alone..

One day I got home and told my wife my intention of not going back to Harlem Hospital because it was not the type of work that I envisioned. I felt a desire and a need to go into private practice. I needed to go into private practice where I could use my organizational skill and God given talent and good bedside skills to help people who desperately needed the help. I informed my wife of my intention of going into private practice. We had discussions about this issue, and my wife was concerned about how I was going to finance an entity such as a medical office and a household..

She was also concerned how we were going to feed our child we were expecting. I was, however, determined to manage it financially especially when we were about to have another mouth to feed. I had during my fellowship and working in the emergency room seen the need for an African American physician in Paterson who could make a difference. I had heard of Drs. Nunez and Short who were gynecologists in town. Dr Short, may he rest in peace, later became a mentor to me. I had met him personally and admired his cool and calm demeanor. I was determined to meet all of them and find out how the private practice environment was in Paterson. I had also been warned that I might have opposition from my fellowship director's group. There was an unwritten rule that no past hematology oncology fellow was welcomed to practice in the Paterson environment, and almost all the fellows left the area as soon as they completed their program. I either did not hear any negative concerns, or I was too determined to be warned about being hindered to practice in the city of Paterson and Passaic County by the same person who helped to train me.

Instead of going back to Harlem, I left for Paterson on Broadway Street hunting for an office space. I came across an empty office on 641 Broadway. The landlady was Mrs. Schwartz. After finding out the rent, I went ahead and signed the contract to rent the office. All I knew was that I was determined to start my private practice and I did not want to look back.

I had made a respectful amount of money whilst I was working in Grenada, so I was able to finance the down payment and several months' rental payment. There and then started my life as a sole practitioner in Paterson.

A lot of my friends told me how hard it was to start a practice de novo, and I was often referred to the fact that there was a reason there were not many African American doctors in town.

I took the challenge and was ready to start afresh and also to take my experience in Grenada as a consultant to help me in the process since I had run a physician specialist consultancy in the island.

My father often told me that no experience, be it good or bad, is ever a loss. "If you look into everything that has gone wrong in your life, there are always positive things that come out of any experience," often said my father.

The statement became a staple in my life, and I believe in that. I said it to myself nobody gave me a chance to get to where I was at this time of my life, but here I was, the cripple my siblings stamped on and ran and the person my father had to carry me on his back to become the first person in my family to go to a university, the second to complete and practice medicine in Mamprugu, the first hematology and oncologist and bone marrow transplant specialist in the whole of the Northern Ghana and one of the very few in the country of Ghana and Africa at large and to one of a few to begin a Bone Marrow transplant establishment is an achievement one could not have imagined.. What else could get me down when I have come from living in a mud hut, ran around naked and barefooted as a child in Bulbia, I said to myself.. The only person who could have scripted my life this way was Allah/God and my ancestors..

I always wanted to make a difference no matter the environment I was in. Looking around Paterson and the Passaic County environ, I knew in my mind that there was a need for me, and it was left to me to fill that void.

Initially I contemplated going back to Ghana, but after my political experience in Grenada, I decided against it. I could still help my people and country more by staying here and practice the high level of medicine I had studied so hard for.

The key entity that influenced me to stay in the United States was the birth of my oldest son on February 13, 1990, just as Mr. Nelson Mandela came out of prison in the then-apartheid South Africa.

I was a proud man and knew I had a mouth to feed. I gave my son the middle name Nelson to represent all the suffering Nelson Mandela had gone through only because he was black and wanted the same rights that was endowed to us by the same maker.. All he wanted to do was to liberate South Africans. I also could no longer pack a bag and travel at a click of a button. Now I had a family, a husband and a proud father of a handsome Mallik Nelson Yamusah. and i was determined to be the best husband and father my wife and son expected me to be. I had a family, and that meant a lot to me.

I armed myself with sheer determination and started my practice as a sole practitioner in the city of Paterson on July 1, 1990. I knew that new walls and barriers were going to come, but at this time i was shielded like a magnetic field or radiation field in a concrete bunker and was ready to go into private practice with enthusiasm and determination.

THE FOURTH PHASE OF ZARA'S CRIPPLED SON'S LIFE

Zara's Crippled Son as a Hematologist and Oncologist in Solo Private Medical Practice in Paterson, N.J. and the Struggles of a Blackman in the American Health Care System.

O n July 1 1990, I opened my private practice in the city of Paterson where I had just completed my hematology and oncology fellowship.

In anticipation of going into the medical business called private medical practice, I had earlier applied for admitting privileges in St. Joseph's Hospital where I had just completed a three year fellowship in Hematology and Oncology, Barnert Hospital in the city of Paterson and in the then Wayne General Hospital in Wayne, N. J that had not yet been purchased by St. Joseph's Hospital. I desired to practice in. St. Joseph's Hospital but the hospital would not even offer me an application for the privileges I was requesting even though I was one of the Emergency room physicians in the same hospital. I was called for an interview in Barnert Hospital where I really wanted to get privileges to admit my patients in private practice. The Chief of Medicine who interviewed me indicated that he had received a letter from my former

Chief of Internal Medicine and Oncology informing him how useless a physician I was.. When Dr. UU said that I chuckled. He then and after that asked me if I was surprised at what Dr. B. had indicated in his assessment letter. He even added that I would have nothing to contribute to the hospital, which was at this time struggling financially to survive.

The chief of medicine in Barnert Hospital had himself worked with me whilst I was a fellow in St. Joseph's Hospital, and in his mind he knew that the assessment given to me by my former director did not match the attributes of the person he himself had personally worked with or heard about in St. Joes. He knew this assessment was rather bizarre, but he was afraid of the reprecussions of him giving me privileges in Barnert and the ramification his decision would affect his position in St. Joseph's where he had privileges in gastroenterology.

At this time there were a lot of rumors in Barnert and St. Joseph's Hospital that Barnert Hospital was going to be closed due to lack of patients as well as a lot of non-insured patients.

I wanted Dr. UU to know that I had heard these rumors too in St. Joseph's Hospital when I was a fellow, and I often said to myself that if presented with an opportunity I was going to do all I could to help the hospital remain open for the African American and Hispanic community who would have an alternative to an institution that had little respect for the population that it claimed it was serving. Some of my patients remembered when blacks and Jews were not allowed into St. Joseph's Hospital. The lack of available health care to the minorities was why Barnert Hospital was established in the first place.

I waited for about a week after my interview, and the final decision was made by Dr. UU that he had decided to give me full privileges in internal medicine, but he was going to put me on a three-month supervised program for the privileges in hematology and oncology. When he called me into the office to give me the' bad' news, he looked as if he was expecting me to be upset. He asked me to sit down and then gave me the options. After this discussion, I could hear my maternal grandmother Amina telling me, "Take what you have now before you expect it to multiply." He indicated to me that since the institution was a Jewish institution and Dr. B was Jewish, a lot of pressure would come down on him if he allowed me to come into the area to compete with Dr. B's group. Indirectly he also was telling me that his own privileges in internal medicine in St. Joseph's Hospital would be at risk since Dr. B was the chief of internal medicine in the same institution.

At this time there was no hematologist and oncologist in this area. All the fellows who were previously trained in St. Joseph's Hospital were often encouraged to move from the area for the fear of being scrutinized and harassed by Dr. B's group, which had Dr. O as the chief of Hematology, Dr. H. as the chief of oncology, and Dr. B, who was an immunologist, as the chief of internal medicine of St. Joseph's Hospital.

From talking to some of the previous fellows and having gone through my Grenada experience, I was more than prepared for what was to come. So I thought.

At this time since my former boss was the chief of medicine and also the de facto chief of hematology and oncology at St. Joseph's Hospital, all my attempts to be given an application form to apply for privileges were never responded to. As the first fellow to do a three-year fellowship, I thought I was entitled to at least an application, and I then had five years to pass my boards. When I was refused an application, I wrote to the president of St. Joseph's Hospital at the time, but I was not surprised at her reaction since the same group that had resented me before was still very active in the hospital. She, however, replied to me that she had no power to request an application for me and that it was left to the discretion of the chief of medicine and the department head who was part and parcel the same person to use his own discretion. It was strange that I could not even get an application in the same institution I had worked so hard for and had received three diplomas showing my ability but was not wanted now by the same institution. This lack of action by the president of the hospital did not surprise me, but I had faith in my god and all my ancestors. My faith in the religious hierarchy had waned to almost the same level I had thought of the devil any way at this point and time.

According to St. Joseph's Hospital's by-laws, as a former fellow, I was entitled to have an application if the principles of democracy and the decency of human life was allowed to take place. I said to myself,

"Haven't you learnt by now that the normal laws of nature have so far not applied in your life?"

I took the Barnert Hospital privileges and met opposition in every hospital in the area.

A lot of my fellowship friends were discouraging me not to take the position. In their mind they thought that I was going to meet the biggest opposition from B's group, and so far, that they knew they had not seen an African American subspecialist having their own office practice in the city of Paterson. Most, if not all, the African American doctors that were working with St. Joseph's Hospital were employed by the hospital. I did not want to be employed by the hospital because I knew I could do better and be successful on my own. Here I remembered when Dr. O told me when I was a fellow during one morning rounds that if I were Jewish, his group would have hired me on the spot. I chuckled but replied politely to him that I was not interested in being hired by anybody no matter my race. He never said a word after that but I thanked him considering me in his thoughts as a competent person who has been disqualified by the color God had given me. I was in no position to change my name to be considered as some people have done in history.

I had in my younger days sold tea and coffee in the lorry station in Walewale to get some few pennies to buy books to go to school, so I knew how to set up an office and initiate a business entity.

I rented an office on Broadway, Paterson, N. J. and started off my practice whilst I was still moonlighting in the St. Joseph's Hospital emergency room where I was refused an application for privileges in internal medicine, hematology, and oncology. I was still good enough to work in the emergency room, but I was not good enough to be given an application for a position as an associate private attending in the department of internal medicine, hematology, and oncology..

My office was hardly furnished, and I decided to start my practice without the fanfare of dressing up every room and other parts of the office. I started by furnishing one room at a time and gradually built it up to the respectable office it is today.

In October 1990, I had become busy enough in the two hospitals in terms of getting consults and self-referred patients. I did not need to work in the emergency room at St. Joseph's Hospital after October

1990, and since my relationship with the hospital had been strained because of their refusal to give me an application as an active member of the medical staff, I decided to end the rest of the relationship since I had no need to work under undesirable conditions. I did not want a token representation as a black man and the more I prayed to God and my deities, the more I was convinced I was doing the right thing.

One advantage that I figured would aid to my success in medical practice was the fact that I was very well-known in the community. I had virtually run the oncology clinic for the three years I was in St. Joseph's Hospital, working as an emergency room physician on my off hours as a fellow (moonlighting) exposed me to the community and finally I had worked in the AIDS(Acquired Immunodeficiency Syndrome) clinic as part of the AIDS management team with Dr. R who was also a nun. It had exposed me to a large population of the Paterson community. Not too many physicians were willing to work in the AIDS clinic in those days, and those of us who were willing to work were often scorned upon.

Both my in-patient admissions and outpatient workload began to increase. I arranged my office hours to cater to the demands of the community. The office was open on Tuesdays, Thursdays, and Saturdays; and the other days were used for in-patient visits, paperwork, and running of the medical practice, which became more businesslike as the years went along. The business of medicine began with the infiltration of Health Maintenance Organizations (HMOs) into the medical establishment in the 1990s.

Expectedly or unexpectedly, I was very heavily scrutinized in all the hospitals I had privileges in. I expected such scrutiny since I was stepping into unchartered waters in the Paterson Township. The minority community consisting of mainly African Americans and Hispanics did not have their own physicians and depended on the mercy of mainly Indian, Arab, Jewish, and other Southeast Asian medical personnel who at times had difficulty extracting their own prejudice from caste systems within their known traditional norms to the U.S. environment, which was mainly divided on socioeconomic grounds. What I was not prepared for was professionals and grown men and women lying and exhibiting hatred, which surpassed what the Ku Klux Klan was capable of without the white robes. I found it

sacrilegious for professional people to lie, cheat, and speak badly about
their colleagues in order to compete and get an upper hand when they
know what they were spreading around was false. Competition can be
healthy if it is achieved honestly. In medicine most of the competition
is often killed by using committees that are often a backbone of
hospital democracy, but it is often used to thwart competition
especially when you have only two or three black Americans in an
institution who often had no representation at all in these committees.
Important committees are often staffed with ethnic and or racial and
religious cannotation.

After about a year in private practice, I did not need to be on call
in the hospital's emergency room. I had enough new patients and
consultation that kept me busy. Within three years, my practice had
picked up, and I needed more examination rooms and space.

Dr. Figueroa, who was retiring then, had an office on the opposite
side of the same street and approached me if I was interested in buying
his office building. After negotiations I bought 634 Broadway in
Paterson, and that was the beginning of my experience in the entity
known as the business of medicine.

I made it a point whenever I went into a new place to go around
and introduce myself to all the shift of nurses on each floor, the
nursing administration, medical records, and emergency room.

As soon as I started in Barnert Hospital as an attending, I noticed
that referrals and consultations were requested and made based on race
and whether the patient had insurance or not.

The same attending that one referred patients would only refer
African American or Hispanic patients to me when they had no
insurance. When they had white Jewish patients or insured African
American or Hispanic patients, they went to Physicians of their like
or their own ethnicity. Most consultations are not made based on
the knowledge or capabilities of the physician and this accounts for
needless deaths in hospitalized patients.

When I was a resident in Englewood Hospital and a fellow in
St. Joseph's Hospital, similar things were going on; but as a fellow,
I saw everybody who came to the hematology and oncology service.
What I did not realize at the time was that medicine even more than
the community was cradled in prejudice. I had some racial issue

throughout my residency and fellowship, but I did not let them bother me. In residency and fellowship the way patients were treated was also racially based.

In my emergency room training in Englewood Hospital, it was always an understanding that most patients who came in as John Does were often young white males who were brought in because of drugs and had a family private physician who did not wish to reveal their family name in order to protect prominent persons or families in the Englewood environs. However, if the patient was an African American or Hispanic, he or she was either identified by their own names or was often labeled as drug addict or alcoholic until their true identity was known. The majority of patients with sickle cell disease who came in painful crises were often labeled as drug addicts and got no attention till the "real" patients were taken care of.

The medico-political environment was very different when I first went into the then Barnert Hospital. The majority of the doctors were Jewish, Arab, Indians, and other Asians. Those of us who were in other groups had to decide which side to affiliate with when medical or geopolitical issues arose.

Hospital Committees were chosen on racial or ethnic lines, and the chairmanship of each committee was chosen and appointed by the president of the medical staff who in turn got his position either on political adherence to one group or belonging to the majority group. These positions were also used to get referrals from physicians who had either started their affiliations with the hospital or had something to lose if they did not give those referrals. Committee chairmanships and president of the medical staff came with its perks. In St. Joseph's Hospital, on the other hand, even though the Indian physicians were well represented, they could not even get a representation in the board of trustees of the hospital.

The most important but subtle perk was in obtaining other referrals for these chairmanship positions. In some cases the chief of internal medicine or chief of surgery was also the president of the medical staff. If a physician was not referring his or her patients to the chairman, no matter how terrible they were in managing the patient, one was often blacklisted and punished in several ways until the physician conformed, was forced to stop admitting patients in that facility, or was forced to move from the area completely so that his or her competitors who conformed to the chairman's rule could get more patients and keep everybody's economic engine rolling. At one time the chief of gastroenterology who had come to Barnert Hospital on a cloud of mismanagement of cases from a nearby institution also became the chief of medicine because at this time there was an Arab majority in Barnert Hospital that had replaced the Jewish majority who had left Paterson in robes for greener pastures in Valley Hospital in Ridgewood, New Jersey, when rumors began to fly about the tentative closure of Barnert Hospital. Despite his tenacious track record that would have disqualified any African American or Hispanic physician, he did not only become the chief of medicine but was also made the chief of gastroenterology because of the said "democratic" process in the hospital. Despite several complications that were brushed under the carpet, he still had a lot of referrals because of fear of the nonconforming physicians being punished. "Give him some consults and shut him up," said a surgeon who was at this time renting him his office, and his rent was not being paid by the chief of medicine. I personally refused to refer my patients to doctors I did not have faith in their management even though I knew that I was going to pay for it with lies, suspensions, and intimidation when heinous crimes were swept under the carpet because one could find Arab representatives as committee chairmen or members. I had worked hard to build a good reputation in the city of Paterson and its environs and was not willing to let my patient get into unnecessary complications. The same thing was happening in St. Joseph's Hospital, but this time it was not only Arabs but Italians who made up the bulk of the teaching staff not because they were more intelligent but because they were well represented in committees and also had their fellow Italians in the management positions in the hospital.

The chief of medicine or surgery controlled who could be on call in the emergency room. The more call days one had, the more the referrals they had to give to the chief. If you were not one of his referral group or you were considered a competitor, then you were not placed on the emergency call list, which made it difficult for young physicians to build their practices. Also, doctors who were neighbors or presumed competitors used the hospital as the playground for economic survival. In my case, because of the demands of the community, I practiced internal medicine, hematology, and oncology. When I first moved into the area, I was warned that my neighbor who practiced endocrinology and internal medicine had been in the location for twenty-five years and he was not going to let another internist to exist hundred yards from his office.

Apparently, word was given to other attendees to warn them on this issue. My neighbor, Dr, L in order to get to me economically, became the chief of medicine and the president of the medical staff twice in order to use the power of his office to initiate an investigation into the use of Heparin for a hematologist and oncologist who used Heparin for central lines(port-caths) and other blood clotting problems and made several illegal attempts to use his position to suspend my privileges in the hospital all because I was having more patients and did not refer my endocrinology cases to him. The maroity Arab and Indian physicians who still wanted domination did not elect Dr. O who was Hispanic and was the Vice- President of the Medical Staff. He was slated to be the next Medical Staff president. A meeting was held by the Arab and Indian physician leaders to present Dr. L as a candidate for the presidency a second time to prevent Dr. O who was a very active surgeon in the hospital from becoming the new president of the medical staff. This meeting was held late in the night in the Doctors launge.

The committees were infiltrated by physicians who did not have patients and had a lot of time to attend committee meetings which they used as a pulpit to get consults from unwilling members of the medical staff. If it happened in Barnert Hospital and St. Joseph's Hospital, I know it is happening in some community hospitals and most medical institutions in this country, which has an impact on the type of medical care that is delivered to the minority population in this country.. Innocent, highly competent black and Hispanic physicians are being destroyed because of the lack of ability for physicians to compete on an equal footing. Minority doctors are not to be loved by patients, and a minority doctor is only considered as competent as others if only one works for an institution. If you are good and your patients love you, it means something is wrong with you and it is the result competing doctors will use their hospital positions to influence the punishment of minority doctors or doctors who are not feeding them.

I actually had the most support from the Jewish groups even though patients were not referred to me except when they had no insurance. They encouraged me to withstand some of the scrutiny my fellow immigrants were bestowing on people they thought were a threat to their economic health and their control of the patient base in the Paterson community. An African American doctor is not to have the majority of the patients in the hospital and was not invited in town, and we were only two when I started off in the department of medicine. Dr. D had gone through worst things. Board certification was made an issue, and almost none of the doctors were legitimately board certified by ABIM in St. Joseph's hospital. Most of them were only board certified on a grandfather's clause within the particular institution they were in. However, even though this was going on, they used board certification as a whipping pulpit knowing very well they were technically in the same group.

As I started my practice, I began to attract a lot of patients; and the more patients one had in the hospital or in the office, the more resentment one had. I did not need to be on call in emergency room to attract patients eventually.

My main mode of advertisement was by oral advertisement by the patients I took care of. As patients who had cancer eventually found their way to me via self-referral, family members came along.

In the hospital initially all consults given to me, whether it was hematology or oncology, were all charity care cases or Medicaid cases. The Medicaid cases never paid anyway, so they were all grouped as my charity care program.

I took care of the patients to the best of my ability as my responsibility to the hospital and the human race. My grandmother's words followed me even into my practice because she often told me when I was young to treat all human beings as God's children, which I did.

I also saw that the same patient who could not pay me had relatives and friends who eventually were referred to me with insurance because of recommendation from the nonpaying patients.

Eventually I realized that the same physician who referred the charity care patients to me often referred their insured patients to doctors of their race, nationality, or religion. I eventually learnt not to take the responsibility alone. When I became the chief of hematology and oncology in Barnert Hospital, the group made an item of understanding that all referrals, whether they had insurance or not, had to be given to the hematology and oncology specialist of the choice of the referral attending so that nobody felt they were being dumped on.

Also around 1995 the HMO (Health Maintenance Organization) era began to creep in when other physicians in the clinics, and the hospital hired specific doctors to take care of the charity care patients rather than relying on the goodwill of doctors and as a societal responsibility.

Obtaining Hospital Medical Privileges in St. Joseph's Hospital, Paterson, N.J.

My practice continued to grow, and the rumors that Barnert Hospital was going to close subsided. The institution seemed like a family unit, and the fifth floor was designated as the oncology floor

In 1995, one day in May, I was standing on the fifth floor, which was the hematology and oncology floor of Barnert Hospital, after I had admitted a number of patients when suddenly I got a tap in the shoulder.

I thought it was one of the nurses playing a joke on me, so I did not turn around. The tap was followed by very familiar voice, which initially stunned me. It was the voice of my former fellowship chief. He asked me if I could walk with him to the side and that he had something he wanted to discuss with me. At this time, still stunned, I could barely move. "What could be happening?" I asked myself. At this point several things began to go through my mind.

It was very shocking because at times I would run into him, and even though I respected and greeted him, he never returned or acknowledged my greetings. In my mind I was very grateful to my boss for giving me an opportunity to become a hematologist and oncologist under him, and despite everything that went through between me and him, I did not feel resentful and would never dream of disrespecting him. My father often said that one does not point ones left hand to his or her own hut where you were born in no matter how big you get. So after hesitation I went with him.

What he told me has startled me up-to-date and made me proud but suspicious.

He told me that he was very proud of me as his former student and for what I had done to help Barnert Hospital and the hematology and oncology program in the hospital.

He indicated that he wanted to give me regional privileges in St. Joseph's Hospital and medical center when he previously would not even give me an application when I first applied after my fellowship training to be an attending in hematology and oncology even though I worked in the emergency room as an attending physician.

He indicated that by getting regional privileges I could transfer patients to St. Joseph's Hospital for both radiation oncology and medical oncology that could not be done in Barnert Hospital. Still stunned but flabbergasted based on prior experience after the discussions, I could not think of any questions to ask him. I thanked him for the conversation and the acknowledgement that I was one of the best fellows if not the best the program has ever had. I could not believe that this was happening even though my mother had told me, "One day your boss will apologise for all you did because you did no wrong. God does not like lies and lies have an ending."

What I did immediately without hesitation was requesting him to send me an application and that I was going to seriously consider his proposal. He wanted to discuss the details later. I finished my rounds and decided to go home. I called my equally stunned wife to inform her of what had just transpired, and I could tell that she was dumbfounded. She wanted to hear more, but I insisted I would speak to her when I got home. My wife has been my friend, my wife, and my sister. She had gone through all these difficulties and sometimes could not understand what was wrong in the medical world. "Don't the other doctors see the injustice in medicine?" she said. Even the doctors who see the unfairness and racism turn a blind eye to it due to selfishness, or they are the ones being helped to gain an upper hand relative to their competitors and "it is not my business syndrome." I went home and discussed this proposal with my wife who could not believe that it happened but advised me to go ahead and fill out the application and send it in if and when it was sent to me. Within one week I got the application, but it was stated that it was only for regional privileges. Since I did not know what the regional privileges entailed, I called the medical secretary at St. Joseph's Hospital to understand the difference between regional privileges and a full attending physician privileges. When I understood the difference, the secretary encouraged me to apply for full attending physician position since I was board certified in internal medicine. I sent in the application and was given privileges in all three specialties.

However, it was not what my former chief wanted, I later found out. He wanted me to get regional privileges so that I could send my patients to St. Joseph's Hospital under his service and the radiation oncology could be fully utilized to boost the bone marrow transplant program, which was almost grinding to a halt under the supervision of his daughter.

When he found out that I had full privileges to admit and to be able to get consultations, he became furious about it, and my life became challenging again even though at this time I did not need consultations in St. Joseph's Hospital to maintain or increase my practice.

I voluntarily refrained from accepting consults in respect to my boss's group and in appreciation of the reversal he had made. I had been called all names in medicine from incompetent to moron even though I was the best fellow in the history of the program. I really felt vindicated when he tapped my shoulder. To me that was an apology, and it was enough to recoup the respect and dignity I had for him.

He also wanted me to be a participant and a contributor of patients to the bone marrow and stem cell program that now had many laminar flow rooms under his supervision and control and now was spearheaded by his daughter who was a hematologist unlike the father. Now I could somehow understand the negativity toward me because he wanted his daughter to run the bone marrow transplant program and not a stranger like me. The daughter, in more than one reason, was not in the same level with me in several aspects., I was not the least envious after I got to know her except that I knew if my father was Dr. B he would not have just given me a position because I was his son. He would have insisted that I had all the academic and personal qualities that was needed to get me the position. In the medical system which race you belong to is very important. If doctors come from outside the U.S. and belong to certain racial groups they do not go through the same scrutiny to get Residency positions. Certain races can often be exempted from taking required examination based on where they come from. Who ever said we were all born equal was definitely dreaming in the world of medicine.. .

Despite my starting the bone marrow transplant program to its fullest capacity and writing all the bone marrow transplant protocols, I was denied privileges in bone marrow transplantation. I did two transplants under his supervision, and since it was not going to make a difference in my professional or economic life, I did not push the issue of pursuing to get full privileges, and I did not want to be supervised because the elements of trust that my patients would be monitored diligently when they were on transplantation was not there. Regaining the trust I had working with confidence in a person I so much respected was the most difficult thing to get back to. I also decided not to take calls in the emergency room because I did not want it to seem as if I was robbing patients from the chief.

Being on call in the emergency room would have meant me being part of the fellowship teaching program, and since he had decided not to involve me in the teaching of the hematology and oncology fellows, I did not deem it wise to stay on call since I had my own patient base.

Most of the physicians on staff could not refer patients to me due to political or ethnic divide, but through self-referrals in town I had a lot of patients from St. Joseph's Hospital. One could not volunteer to teach in the internal medicine residency or hematology/oncology fellowship program because the hospital had assigned certain doctors to take on the teaching task. I considered it an Italian group since only certain ethnic groups of doctors were allowed to participate in the teaching program and were paid to do it. In my residency and fellowship programs, I was used to interacting with all the physicians and teaching positions were voluntary so that trainees could get a wide scope of different styles of practicing medicine.

One of the aspects of medicine that will change in a negative way in small community teaching institutions is the lack of participation of varying medical doctors teaching the fellows, residents, and students. Apparently it has been a change during the HMO era when everybody was paid even to teach on rounds and nobody taught out of the love of the profession or the genuine love for teaching. Even where one interacted with residents or fellows who had a problem or needed direction one's attempt to help is often considered interference. The hospital had assigned physicians who were not necessarily the best at what they did or the best at bedside teaching but made sure positions were made up of friends of ethnic divide and physicians who would only concur with the norm. To me this impacted on the quality of teaching and the variety of patient care a resident or fellow is engaged or exposed to. When I was a fellow, we had students from schools like St. George's University. My attending, not remembering that it was my alma mater, told me not to spend too much time with the students or residents because they became equals and could compete with American-trained doctors when they passed their internal medicine boards.

It was an alarming comment, but it was the truth because of the quality of teachers they had teaching.

Due to the lack of cultural diversity, we had African Americans, Hispanics, and other minority patients who came in with medical problems that could not be explained without involving the cultural niche in history taking. There was an incidence when a Ghanaian male was admitted through the emergency room to another physician's service. He kept telling the resident that somebody cast 'juju' on him, and as a result, he was poisoned. That is why he was bleeding from his mouth. The next thing one noticed was an order for serum and urine toxicology because the resident thought he was hallucinating from a drug addiction. It was not realized that in Ghana or in most African and some Caribbean countries and states like Louisiana nobody dies of a disease process. The impact of the process of how other persons may do harm to their friends or enemies or can cast voodoo or juju on their fellow humans cannot be understated.

Cultures have a unique tendency to blame human frailties or frailties for all medical conditions, and if one cannot decipher that aspect of history taking and focus on the realistic ones, one would be led to a wrong diagnosis. After I spoke to the gentleman and took a defined history based on Ghanaian culture, this young man was helped. This began a storm or wave of discussions the next day, and I was verbally told I could not teach the residents since I was not a member of the teaching staff who were either grandfathered board certified or none at all.

It is often thought to medical students, residents, and fellows how important history taking is. However, if an entity that varies from culture to culture has no representation at the attending level even though majority of the patients are African Americans or Hispanics, then the system is not being fair to the population they purport to serve. In St. Joseph's this is a constant hindrance from private African American or black attending to participate in the process unless one is hired by the institution and make one person a representation of all Negroid people. It is difficult in a democratic country to allow minorities in institutions such as a hospital not because the minorities do not apply or do not qualify but solely because of their skin pigmentation. Often in replacement of the real reasons of not hiring minorities often includes we cannot find qualified minorities or they perfect the lies and innuendoes to keep people out of the so-called religious or private institutions.

In Barnert Hospital as in St. Joseph's Hospital several investigations were carried out by the administration and other physicians about inappropriate use of cardiac catheterization facilities on my patients even though I was not a cardiologist. At the time of the investigations, nobody informed us about the reason for such investigations. It was several years later that it was brought to my attention that the institutions wanted to correlate history taking and findings on cardiac catheterization to see if the procedure was done unnecessarily on African American and hospital patients. They correlated nurse history taking with regard to chest pains and cardiac catheterization results. It was a year later that I learnt that such a study was carried out without the knowledge of the cardiologist that I had referred the patients or myself. The results were only ignored after they found that the history obtained correlated with coronary artery syndrome and also on catheterization corresponded with vessel disease, and also because it did not give the institutions the results they desired to hang my neck. Apparently my history taking was better than that of the nurses and first-year residents! Whew!!!I had nothing to hide about my capabilities, and also as a kid I always had a good penmanship, which made it easier for persons to read my handwriting. The scrutiny of my charts was being done in St. Joseph's and Barnert Hospital not to make me improve but so that any mistakes could be used against me.

I was also adamant to help the institution as to the cultural divide that existed and still exists today in a culturally mosaic town.

For example, if one should ask a Jamaican patient the Anglo-Saxon way if they had chest pains, they immediately would clamp down and become reluctant to go with you with an honest interview. But if you ask a Jamaican about their "gas" and characteristics of their gas and then direct your questions in the cardiac direction, one would likely illicit cardiac pathology. Most South Americans and people from the Caribbean have hesitations about discussing or even calling the word "cancer," but if one educates the family and explains to them why I cannot treat a patient without their knowledge, they will with draw their request of treating their relative without their knowledge. One basic problem I noticed during my residency and fellowship years was the subtle discrimination that went on in medicine and how it was left untouched. I had attendings who would not touch a patient because they were dirty. I would stand there and wonder because we just came out from an equally dirty white lady and he had no problem examining that patient. When it came to explaining the condition to the patients, it was always the African American and Hispanic patient who was hardly spoken to because they cannot understand. Most of the time on rounds, one could see how the demeanor of the attending would change as we went from one race to the other. I strongly believe that if a patient cannot rely on their caretakers for respect, then what kind of health care are we giving? On rounds it was the African Americans that one would not disturb because they are sleeping when, in fact, they were wide awake. It was the same group who could not understand. It was children of African Americans who had sickle cell who came in, in painful crises who was often called a junkie.

By involving minority participation in the teaching programs, it will not only aid the medical students, residents, and fellows in having more understanding of a disease process that we the medical society has aided and abetted to make the sickle cell patients into drug junkies. They are often made to stay in pain and made jokes of and finally given a narcotic injection and sent home without his disease process being thought of more diligently before the patient is sent home only to come back in a few hours and will now be admitted and left alone to sleep out the effects of his narcotic injection. It was the same African American except when you were a politician who often had their complaints of subpar treatment that was ignored. If a Caucasian called on the call bell, everyone would be running helter-skelter to satisfy the patient. The bigotry is not limited to doctors only or to white workers only, but also the same black nurses and home health aides are even worst to their kind. We cannot take care of people when we think they are less human; and the health care system has to wake up and realize that no doctor, nurse, or nursing assistants wants to be called a racist, yet we practice it every day. We can mandate people to attend cultural and diversity classes, but as we saw during the civil rights era, unless the hierarchy wakes up and realizes medicine is still a century behind in treating all as equals in this country, the disparity in medical care that is often attributed to everthing but racism will continue to cause systemic failures in the system. Medicine should learn how to respect one's cultural or religious beliefs, and incorporate it into the art of healing that we have dedicated our lives to uphold. By involving minority participation in the teaching programs, it will not only make the students, residents, or fellows better and culturally sensitive but would make them excellent physicians for all persons especially in a multicultural environment like the city of Paterson. I came out of fellowship vowing not to follow the same prejudicial pathway I was taught. I have treated all my patients with respect and dignity. My bedside acumen is unbeatable, and I have been very successful. I have demanded respect from all consultants, nurses and nursing assistants in hospitals that I have had medical privileges for my patients. Everybody in my treatment team knows what I demand for all my patients, and they adhere to that code. They are encouraged to answer to questions no matter who the patients are and no matter their cultural background. When Barnert Hospital was labeled as a bad hospital, my patient loved it because of the standard set about the care of my patient. For example if a white old lady seeks help in the hospital the staff will move fast to assist her but if an equally old black lady rings her room's bell for assistance, you often hear the aide and/or nurse screaming at the poor lady or ignoring the call completely until a family member intervenes. In st. Joseph's and Banert Hospitals equally addicted white and black young males were often metted different treatment and the black patient often ended up with abuse and little care. The reason for this disparity in care is how the administration or Physician and nursing administrations react in response to the two groups. A white patient complaining about in issue often got the employee fired or disciplained and there was no similar consquencies when it involved the black patient. If the set up of the system was such that the hospital metted the same or some form of punishment when ever complaints of similar nature was made we would not have disparity in care. In most instituitions the black or Hispanic patient is more likely to end up with decubital ulcers than a similar white patient irrelevant of their insurance status . The African American patient tends to have more co-morbid problems and is often discharged home hurriedly when the system knows how difficult it is to get home care services to them in our big cties. Home care services are non-existent in cities like Paterson after s.oop.m. The African Amwerican stroke patient was often not referred to the Kessler Institute when I started my private practice. In most cases, the social workers also steamlined where to send patients of certain ethnic groups to.. It was not unusual for a social worker to indicate to me that there were no beds in Kessler Institute when they had not even considered sending the patient to that institution in the first place.. There is a system wide unequal treatment when it comes to the healthcare in this country. It is a topic the whole system will not even accept discrimination is happening in all aspects of medicine. It is ofen agreed upon that there is disparity in the care of blacks when compared to whites. What medicine will not agree is that one of the main causes of this disparity is a form of racism. Until the system accepts that there is a problem, we will continue to see a spiraling increase in healthcare cost in a system that has been skewed since the time of slavery and has barely changed because we are made to pretend that things will change only when they are left alone. I have come up in life living and still feels the subtle effects of racism. No human being should belong to the low echelon in life because we are are all God's children. We often demand the love and peace from God, yet we hate our neighbor or the sick patient whose only reason for being in the hospital is because they are ill and black or Hispanic..

Teaching (Non-private) and Non-teaching (private) patients: The role of the Black and Hispanic patient and how Hospital politics influences their care.

The fact that I admitted most of my patients as "private" or "nonteaching" was also an unacceptable element to the administration even though it was the right of my patients and my responsibility as an attending physician to decide which of my patients had pathology that could be used for teaching the medical students, Resident and fellows..

For persons who do not understand the terms "private" (nonteaching) or "non-private" (teaching) patients, it can be explained this way. When a patient is admitted to a hospital, the patient is often considered whether they have insurance, no insurance; have a private medical attending on staff or not.. The insured patients are often admitted to private attending who would manage the patient under his or her care. The non-private patients which make up the bulk of the patients used for teaching students, residents, and fellows—are either insured or noninsured. Most African American and Hispanic patients make up the bulk of the teaching programs in most teaching institutions in America from whom students, residents, and fellows learn. I personally did not see anything wrong with my patients being admitted to teaching solely because they were African American or Hispanic as long as my patient was respected and consented to being used for teaching. Most patients were never consulted and actually had no choice as to their participation in teaching activities in the hospital. Apparently the authorities of St. Joseph's Hospital were watching without my knowledge whilst I was admitting patients since ninety-five percent of my patients were either African American or Hispanic Americans. What I wanted to do was to strike a conversation as to how a minority doctor felt about the care given to minority patients especially the African Americans and Hispanics who made up the bulk of the teaching service and who were more likely not to be admitted as private whether they had medical insurance or not through the emergency room.

Several changes had taken place from 1999 in both St. Joseph's and Barnert Hospital, so I did not know and had never met the new chief of medicine in St. Joseph's Hospital. I was, however, very disappointed as to how we finally got to meet and the circumstances that led to our meeting. On two occasions I had an altercation with a fellow physician who I was later to learn was the chief of medicine. I had come to the garage of St. Joseph's Hospital to pack my car at the designated "doctors only" portion of the garage. The security guards by now knew who I was, and so they waved me to park at a spot, which I did. Immediately I stepped out of my car, a tall almost grayish white male walked up toward me; and in his exact words, he said, "This is a parking space for doctors only. Why did you park there?" I proceeded to ask him if he was a parking attendant, but something held me back. Not knowing who he was, I said to him that I was one of the attending physicians on staff in St. Joseph's Hospital. He introduced himself as Dr. M and proceeded to walk away.

After I introduced myself and got to know him for the first time, he did not say a word to me or apologize for taking me to be security guard in his mind.

I, in fact, took my identification badge showing him that we were in the same department. I offered my hand, but he did not replicate the gesture. I said to myself that he knew who I was since he had taken over from my former boss as the chief of medicine. After he refused to shake my hand for the fear that probably I was going to make his hands black or for whatever reason, I quickly told him I had to go and I left. I did not think this encounter was intentional, and if it was an intentional one, then it was very well calculated.

Approximately six weeks later at about the same spot, the same thing happened. Immediately when I came out of my car, he asked me for my identification as a physician. Dr. M had forgotten he had met me six weeks earlier at almost the same spot

I showed him my badge again and also called my name again to him. I became perplexed why the chief of medicine had begun to work in the garage and was so forgetful that he could not remember us meeting previously.. He again left without a word after identifying himself. The third time he walked up to me and said, "So you are Dr. Yamusah." I concurred and acknowledged him by saying, "How are you today, Dr. M?" He then proceeded to indicate to me that it had come to his knowledge that I only admitted my patients as private and he wanted me to desist the practice because it was influencing the population base of African American and Hispanic patients who were increasingly refusing to participate in the teaching program. He also indicated they were demanding that they did not want to be used as guinea pigs and wanted to be treated better. What is wrong with their thought, I asked.

I proceeded to ask him if he wanted to know why I made my patients private. He quickly turned his head away from me and told me that he did not want to hear anything on my behalf but warned me if I did not stop the practice of admitting my patients as private, he was going to make my life miserable. I wanted to call the security guard to witness this third episode, but I thought of the vulnerability of a young Hispanic male who was the attendant then becoming a witness. I reasoned that if I am a physician and I could be harassed this way, how could I engage a minority security guard. Afterward I left to complete my rounds. If he had listened to me, I would have expressed to him that because of the lack of respect African American and Hispanic patients were getting from the higher up in the administration, it was influencing the way the students, residents, and fellows acted and treated the same population that was used as tools to teach them. I would have told him that I remembered when I was a fellow most white patients even if they had no insurance were admitted as private patients not only in St. Joseph's Hospital but also in Englewood Hospital where I trained. I wanted to tell him how histories of service patients were read to the hearing of everybody on the floors when residents were on their rounds with no regard to the patient's privacy.

Patients were not asked before their participation in teaching and were not given an option not to participate. Patients were treated as investigative specimen rather than a respected human being with full rights and dignity. Patients were segregated on floors not only on disease entity but also based on race. Most African Americans and Hispanics who were the bulk of the teaching floor, when they were HIV positive, were placed on one floor, the fifth floor but patients who were nonteaching patients in this case were predominantly white patients even though they had the same diagnosis could be placed on any floor the attending physician requested or desired

I would have also told him how some patients came up and never saw a licensed doctor's supervision until they were discharged by residents. I was ready to help to make the teaching program even better and inclusive. After all, St. Joseph's Hospital was where I trained as a fellow and all these entities had existed for many years prior to my training there and probably still exist after my absence and I doubt if it has changed today. As a fellow, one could not effectively help in the changes of some of the pitfalls even though these pitfalls were shortcoming not in St. Joseph's Hospital alone but in all institutions that had teaching programs. Medicine seems to be years behind the civil rights movements and still lacks representation in the minority groups that make up the bulk of the teaching program.

Physicians who come from countries that practiced or had caste systems and big disparity between the "have" and the "have-nots" do not think a problem exists because the same thing was going on in their own communities. The few African American and Hispanic physicians, even though they see and feel these disparities, often pretend they did not exist or are afraid of harassments, demotions, and professional lies that are used to demonize them. They turn a blind eye to these problems in outright fear. Also, when a physician is under scrutiny because he has more patients than others or other non-justifiable reasons, the cost of trying to defend oneself is often so exorbitant that most physicians cannot afford to hire lawyers who often follow the same racial tactics to defend them. The best solution is usually to shut one's mouth, partially close one's eyes enough so that one can walk away without seeing the glowing problems of racial injustice they are looking down on.

As a resident in Englewood Hospital, even these disparities occurred with how residents were perceived. On certain religious days, members of certain religious groups were excused from work whilst others were made to cover for the fortunate or privileged groups. Most of the residents often closed their eyes and ears and did the work without complaining because the repercussions of such complaints were indirect punishment to the residents. Upon coming out of residency and fellowship and as an attending in an institution that was thought could do better morally especially in a catholic institution contrary to all the experience with that institution I still felt that somethings could be done to steer the institution out of its traditional stand of racism. Since the chief of medicine did not think that as a black man I could be a doctor to park in the physician parking space; I wondered if one could get anywhere trying to help make some changes. It was not only the chief of medicine alone who often saw a black man as an element of fear, threat, and intimidation; but it is a whole societal issue that a democratic country finds itself preaching to the rest of the world what it cannot practice itself as seen with the string of unwarranted deaths of blacks in the hands of the same institution which is supposed to protect them.. In that light, as a black doctor I am not often recognized as such but often given other titles such as the orderly, the instrument technician and the clerk in every institution i have worked as a black man. . Requested not to park in a doctor's designated parking lot was not only strange for a professional who headed a program in a predominantly African American and Hispanic American area but insinuated that as a black man I could not be a doctor. I wondered if I could get anywhere if he had stopped to have a discussion with me. In my mind he had no intention to understand the direction I was coming from but was only interested in throwing allegations against me as an instruments to get me out of the hospital. After my presence, the chief of pathology who was an African American had her office door padlocked with the insignia that she did not fit the direction in which the hospital was going, and the most popular person and showcase African American who was also the chief of emergency services that I had worked under suddenly found out that he did not fit the agenda after certain changes were made in St. Joseph's Hospital

Several other items happened that I thought were irrelevant, but the nursing staff would tell me that certain medical staff personnel were looking into my charts. There were times I would come to carry out my rounds on my patients, and their charts would be mixed up. The nursing staff who were very concerned about some of the unprofessional behavior that was going on would inform me. Most of the copying of my charts took place at 5:00 p.m. when the quality management would be leaving, and if one came at a later time to write notes, then I was accused of postdating my notes.

Quality Care Management, Hospital Committees, the Hospital administration, the Black Doctor, the Black patient and institutional racism in American Health Care.

Quality management tools were made in order to assure the practice of good medicine and the extension of what is called quality management to patients. This quality management became a political tool to be used by medical groups to satisfy their disdain for certain groups especially physicians who were perceived to be popular in the community or had more patients than other physicians. One was required to attend conferences and meetings, but when one participated, there were doctor police officers who would document what notes were written or not. Quality management was instituted to control hospital costs, ensure the delivery of quality medicine, and boost the economic survival of hospitals. Up-to-date no institution with a quality management team can show that their quality management team has helped reduce cost. If that was not the case, why are so many hospitals closing down? What actually happened was bloated salaries for quality care teams and the withdrawal of nurses who were experienced from the bedside. . Physicians who were members of the quality care teams but had medical practices in the same community used quality management as their pulpit to do harm to physicians they did not like or were competing with in the community. The quality management teams joined to boost the medical teams that thought their existence in the hospital was a necessary entity and those that thought that a bureaucracy had been built to retaliate against popular doctors or doctors who brought in patients into an institution.

A lot of hospitals including my dear Barnert Hospital have closed despite the fact that they had quality management teams that bloated budgets and at the long run participated in sucking the economic health out of the institution

One lawyer asked me why an institution in which I was the dominant physician would not be appreciative to me in order for more patients to be brought in. The answer was that the physician bringing in the patients to the hospital did not fit in the right ethnicity. I was chastised for giving good care to the population they indicated they were representing. Quality management programs did not monitor complications caused by heads of department and their favorite physicians, but God forbade that you were out of their political stratosphere or ethnic group one would be found in default of entities that were made up or one did not know existed.

Hospital management teams were not business minded. The administration and administrative politicians would recommend and carry out projects that were solely based on whose name plate was to be placed on which building. For example, in the late 1990s there was a debate in the then Barnert Hospital whether to modernize the surgical suites, which would amount to millions of dollars, which the institution that depended on charity care dollars from the state did not have. When it was brought ahead for discussion, even the CEO and certain physicians were not in support of it, and I was one of them. The main reason I did not support the project was because none of the politically inclined surgeons brought any of their own or the same-day surgeries to Barnert Hospital. They actually took some of the patients who were seen in the surgical, breast, or gynecology clinics and transferred them to hospitals such as Valley or Hackensack hospitals;

and they did this out of pride. Barnert Hospital and Patersonians did not deserve patients being brought to their environs to be taken care of, yet these same physicians headed departments and projects where they were being paid heavily by the hospital. By the time the hospital got the charity care dollars, there was nothing left to uplift the hospital. Doctors whose livelihood depended on the institution had nothing good to say about Barnert Hospital. Physicians even denied they had offices in Paterson even though all their well-earned money was from Paterson.

When one opposed the using of multimillion dollars to renovate an entity that had no committed surgeons, urologists, etc., to use the surgical suites based mainly on the economic viability of the institution, one became an enemy not only to his colleagues but also to the board of trustees who had members who also had side economic interests on these projects. What eventually happened was that Barnert Hospital, in not thinking properly of how funds were used, renovated a four-million-dollar surgical suite that stood like a camel in the middle of the Sahara Desert without a camel driver to direct it. The hospital eventually closed out of financial mismanagement, and the same people who wanted these projects turned around and blamed other people for the woes of the hospital.

In any institution the type of leadership is an important entity in order for that institution to run efficiently. Barnert Hospital throughout the 1990s had numerous CEOs who worked diligently to keep the *institution* afloat. It was finally decided that the institution should have its first and only female CEO. This female CEO was very much known to the medical staff since she was previously the medical staff officer at one time. After she was elected or appointed, certain elements of the medical staff could not stand the idea that a female CEO would lead them. Their ethnic or religious upbringing did not induce them into having a female CEO. Whatever she did— and most of her policies were for the betterment of the hospital— was vehemently opposed. There were certain ethnic groups who felt that their cultural and religious beliefs were more important than the good of the institution. Every effort was made to eventually dismiss the CEO when the giant albatross was built and nobody used it. What was so hypocritical was the fact that the same physicians who had disdain for the female CEO were the same persons who were carrying fake petitions for her reinstatement when they worked diligently to kick her out, on the same day her father died.. After she left, there was a downward spiral to the coffers of the institution because subsequent administrations came in and had no control of the medical hierarchy who were not the admitting doctors. The administration carried out projects they wanted but as long as they did anything the physician management wanted. There was a sense of cohesiveness that was closed solely on the hospital materials and monetary entities being passed from one point to the other. Emergency room calls became a lucrative business. Only certain ethnic groups could get calls because of the ethnicities of the chief of the departments who was now an Arab after the Jewish physician left in anticipation of the closure of the hospital. The ensuing chaos and monetary mismanagement led to the hospital's closure.

Another case in point where there was disagreement between the administration executives and the medical staff was when it was decided that a family medicine residency program would help bring money to the hospital. In the nearby St. Joseph's Hospital, teaching programs and fellowships were being closed. What are we doing to get a residency program? Without fanfare we had a family medicine residency program that was not planned and ending up not helping the institution or the residents who were brought into the program. They had two chiefs who virtually did nothing. Majority of the residents were African Americans, and it was my fear that these residents did not see what lay in front of their future because there was really no program. One day I came on the floor, and all five of the residents were waiting for me to go on rounds with my patients. I made myself available to them because they were minority students like I was, and I knew how society would treat them if they were not well prepared for the real world. I was not chosen as a member of the residency staff, but my services were required. However, every meeting or food gathering place, one would see the chief. Some of the residents began to come to me for help. In my zest to help, I would approach the CEO about how the residents did not have a set program.

Eventually, after I saw that the so-called chief of the program thought that a threat had been presented to him, I completely withdrew from the program. The residents had no calls and no supervisors, and residents came as they wished. The monies that were expected to arise from the school of osteopathic medicine and the federal Medicare program did not materialize, but the hospital was paying huge salaries for teachers and program doctors who had no idea how to run a program. The residency program eventually died with the hospital. Had somebody listened and observed, they would have noticed that Barnert Hospital was not mentally or morally capable of handling the program and should not have been given that opportunity.

Pep projects are and will continue to lead to closing of a lot of institutions unless there is an equitable debate, research, and the acceptance and respect of the minority in these institutions. More hospitals will fail, and the cost of medicine, which is the main goal of reducing cost, will only remain a dream no matter how we attempt to reframe the medical care system.

Institutions want everything to themselves. No institution wants to share an MRI machine, PET/CT scanner, and joint programs. By institutions wanting to maintain their own independence at any cost, economic laws will have no respect, and more institutions will collapse, and the cost of medicine will continue to spiral out of place in the hard economic times we are in.

In my case the close scrutiny made me not too concerned about somebody looking at how I was managing my patients because I took diligent and respectful care of my patients and my clinical medical knowledge and bedside acumen is unbeatable.

What I was not prepared for was the lies and cheating that professional people could generate in a Catholic religious institution with members of the clergy always available for patients who needed help. Personally I thought the physician hierarchy and some of the political clergy needed help too. I often suggested the Virgin Mary should help our medical administration so that nobody had to lie, cheat, and harm another physician to rise up the political ladder in the institution. These tactics have destroyed not only minority physicians but also well-meaning doctors who are driven through human frailties to drink alcohol, do drugs, and succumb to heavenly pressures.

Most of the time on my office days, I often did my hospital rounds late in the night. During the rounds all patients were seen first and I then sat down and completed my progress notes. This was a practice i developed with numerous other doctors who formed a quasi group of nightclub physicians. These doctors included Dr. K, Dr. N, and many other doctors. When I came on these hours, I would make sure I saw my patients before sitting down to write my notes. In time of emergencies, I would be in the hospital till about 2:00 a.m. Apparently I was being monitored in this group, and the chief of medicine began to accuse me ofpost-documentation and came out with charts of copies that were erroneous to me. One day Dr. M, who now recognized me, called me to accuse me of post-documentation. In all my years as a private Medical Attending I was never brought up before a committee for mismanagement, morbidity or mortality. I took care of my patients very well, and I was one of the busiest doctors in both hospitals. But somewhere I knew something will be concocted to try to discredit my clean image. It ended up that Dr. M later was found not to have a license to practice medicine in New Jersey yet did not only head a program he had no business running but sat in judgement of people who were licensed and qualified than he did. He was unceremoniously let go when the truth came out. My mother often says that a lie cannot lay low for too long because God does not love ugly and the truth eventually comes out irrespective of the time period. People sit in judgement of others even though they hide under the banner of being the privileged in the field of medicine. They make up things to destroy people who have worked so hard to achieve what they have only to end up being destroyed by a system in medicine where one cannot tell the truth any more. If one doesnot conform to the lies cheating and the plain racism that goes on one is not a comformist and one ends up being destroyed whilst the real criminals hide under suits and cloak the grand dragon of the Klu klux kan will not dare wear..

I was accused of post-documentation and length-of-stay issues even though I was dealing with some of the very sick and terminally ill patiens whom at times I was forced to discharge them. All these investigaions were spear headed by Dr, L whose office was a hundred yards from mine who used his friends in St. Joeeph's Hospital and in Barnert Hospital where he was now the President of the Medical Staff to stifle my practice., When asked for the proof of what financial loss the hospital incurred nobody could come out with the answer. In most of these institutions, . Physicians are often appointed by the head of the Department committees to make judgments against their competitors in violation of U.S. anti-trust laws. The president of the medical staff in Barnert Hospital often filled all key committees with his like or his friends in order to do harm to unwilling physicians or competitors. There were cases in which certain physicians were often reported to the state health authorities whilst real crimes such as gastric perforations and punctured lungs went unreported. Who cares about the hospital by-laws? It is a document of laws to benefit which ethnic group was in the majority in the hospital at that time. Sometimes young doctors who come into institutions that other physicians think will surpass them often start to put traps on the road for those physicians so that they will be frustrated and finally either move or join the same team in order to stop the competition. When I was a resident in Englewood, I remember what Dr. R, who was the only active African American physician on the medical staff, told me. He was one of three black attending's in that hospital, and I doubt if it has changed over the years. He told me that all my smiles would disappear if I went into private practice. He said that the same attending, physicians working with me now would try to bar me from getting privileges after I finished my Resdency program. He told me about some of the sabotaging and lies he had to go through that resulted in involving himself with alcohol. "They will do everything to destroy you because you will be a good physician in private practice." I often heard about some of the physicians expressing bad words about him anytime he admitted a patient. How can human beings be so cruel to another who did not choose for God to give him a black skin? As a resident I could not understand all that was going on. All the bitterness, scrutiny, and mental abuse resulted in Dr. R's demise. The black and Hispanic society that was the reason for all this scrutiny did not help Dr. R's fight with the establishment. The African American and Hispanic people and their politicians do not support their own because they often think that the physician can handle it. Once the black and Hispanic politicians are given private rooms in a hospital they do not see what their electorate is /are going through and frankly do not think they care, Mr. MK who was the photographer when he took pictures of me when I was running the first Bone Marrow Tansplantation in st. Josephs Hospital told me in a meeting in Paterson city hall that St, Joseph's hospital did not want to give me privileges not because I was not qualified but because i did not belong to the Italian mafia. He made this statement whilst he was a Paterson Council man and an Ombusman of St. Joseph's Hospita where he was also being paid and still fulfilled a position as a public official of the patients whose lifes I was saving.

In the future, what needs to be done to protect good, capable, and young physicians, be they minorities or not, should be addressed in such a way that physicians or their related groups, either with direct or indirect group affiliations, should not be allowed to sit in judgment of any physician they want their economic demise so that they can be protected from predators. The partners of anybody in authority who solicits for consult should also be exempted. Any threats or illegal activities that will threaten the life of another physician should have law enforcement involved and not be brushed under the administrations broom as is usually done. My office and office door was vandalized a number of times when a physician lost his bid to purchase my current office ahead of me.. An independent physician body should be made on a district or regional level to oversee any action taken against a physician before any disciplinary action is taken against a physician to prevent anti-competitive schemes, racism and fraud. Diversity schemes should also be set up to monitor how minority patients who make up the majority of the teaching patients are treated. It is not just enough to sign a consent form but what is explained to innocent patients before they consent to procedures and experimental protocols is equally important. It is sad that patients from Saudi Arabia and other countries can come to St. Joseph'sjoseph's Hospital and get the best of care. The doctors are often paid for their services whilst charity care is made to pay the Hospital bills when citizens cannot be accorded the same care in their own environment. Children can be brought into this country to get care to show the charity nature of institutions when there are the same poor and indigent are left running from Medicaid clinic to another and whom no real doctor will even touch them and are left to the mercy of students and interns who are often thought the same tricks and attitude towards the same people they used to learn.

A lot of innocent and well-trained physicians have been damaged and destroyed by this negative use of the medical establishment because the medical system is in disarray. There is no source for official complaint without having to spend thousands and thousands of dollars getting attorneys who do not do anything to help the physician.. Most young physicians do not have the income to fight these issues, so they either move from one city to another or from state to state sometimes in fear of their lives from competitors who sit in judgment in committees purposely to destroy capable and excellent doctors. Maybe a consideration should be given in the midst of the health care bill where a legal institute can be established that can be used by both feuding parties to discuss discord before arbitrary conclusions can be made to defame others or threaten another physician's existence and also before any action is taken on any sacrificial physician lamb.

In Barnert Hospital, the some issue was going on. There had been a series of changes in the administrations due to poor performance of the hospital economically, yet the hospital had no problem paying physicians and non-physicians to be on call in the emergency room and surgical calls and getting paid using the charity care dollars, which were meant to be used for improvements in the quality of care of the hospital. Majority of the private physicians did not bring their private patients to Barnert Hospital because their patients were too good, rich, or non-minority; and they did not want to be associated with a hospital in Paterson whilst the attending physician depended hand and foot on the hospital's resources and governmental monies to enrich each other.. The president or department heads and chiefs often put up ego-seeking programs such as autistic care programs, breast care centers and diabetic management programs, which helped no patients except the managers who were handsomely paid. Economic entities such as the hyperbaric wound care program and the sleep laboratory programs, which were initially successful programs and run very well by the establishment directors, due to personal jealousy among physicians then became money-losing entities and further drained the economy of an already-struggling institution The administration had infiltrated itself with the same selfish physicians that they were supposed to watch. The administration put up programs like refurbishing a multi-million dollar surgical suite which was solely to please the physician leadership and hierarchy when they well knew no surgeons were committed to the institutions and did not admit their private patients or bring their private patients for any outpatient surgical procedure The multimillion dollar "giant" was built, but it was hardly used until the hospital closed due to mismanagement and not due to lack of insured patients as was portrayed by the media.

After 2000 I concentrated all my efforts in Barnert Hospital and improved my office to eventually be self-sufficient. Private medical practice is what I always wanted to do, and it has been my best endeavor. It has not only been challenging from the patient's point of view but also from an economic standpoint. It has also enabled me to understand the different cultures and medical problems from all corners of the world because the city of Paterson is a mosaic of cultures. I have an equal amount of African American and Hispanic patients and a minority white patient base, and my patients have often brought joy and tremendous amount of learning and satisfaction to me. They have made medicine to be what I expected. It is all about the human being. We came to this world alike, and we will leave this world to go back to our next world the same way we came into this world no matter our religious, racial or ethnic convictions. The Kantonsi tribe symbolizes the Placenta as a white cloth and at the end of life we are buried with only the white cloth to symbolize our return to our beginning. We cannot carry hatred or gold into the next world so we have to be good to each other.

The medical profession has to think and come out of the box. The isolation of the profession to religious, racial, color, ethnic, bigotry dominants affects the quality of medical care. A physician who is in an environment that they are made to feel they do not belong often results in increase in cost and suspicion. The minority physicians are often scrutinized not because they are not good or excellent physicians, but they are not an accepted group unless they are employed so that any mistake, be they human or nonhuman, can be created to make the institution very uncomfortable for the minority doctors to keep jumping from one institution to the next or move from one part of the country to the next. Even though cities like Newark and Paterson are inhabited by African Americans and Hispanics, barely are these groups represented in the hospitals in those areas as private physicians.. These physicians are hindered from getting application forms or from attaining privileges because the population that the hospital service would tend to go to their own kind who can understand their culture and behavior patterns. Physicians have been known to refuse other physician privileges in a hospital based on fear of the popularity of the physicians in the community. In the era of the Hospitalist the hospitals now have their own and thwarts competition by not giving popular physicians in the community privileges so that they will have enough private patients to supplement and pay their hospitalist.. They stretch the truth and defame other physicians and use character assassination to cover the unjust activities that are perpetuated in these institutions. Even though "minority" doctors in the medical profession make up a small percentage of the profession, the rate of drug dependence, alcohol abuse, and psychological ailments and industry-related suicides are more predominant in that minority group. They are in a profession who will do anything including lying and cheating to make the deprived and abused physician look not only as a victim but even become the victim.

When the minority doctors cannot get help, they often fall to the legal system, which is no better in the way they treat their minority clients. Physicians have been known to move from certain towns or districts because they do not have enough capital to fight legal battles that could simply have been solved if there was a mechanism the disadvantaged physician could be heard. When a damaged physician has to pay five hundred dollars an hour to defend one's credibility and if you do not have funds at any stage of your defense, you can be dropped because of lack of money; it is easier for the physician to keep moving from one hot zone to the other until they are comfortable. This comfort almost always comes from the federal government, the military, and the army. They may end up volunteering to fight in wars because they are fighting silent wars in their hospital environment anyway..

Post Closure of Barnert Hospital, Hospital Monopoly and the Blackballing of Community physicians.

For several years the Hospital did well and was able to stay open. In 1990 when i first became one of the few Black physicians it was a nice place. It was a place where my hope for the best care of the minorities in Paterson could be realized. I walked into the hospital to see a divided camp of physicians. The majority of the physicians was Jewish followed by Asian Indians and a minority Arab population. The hospital at the time only supplied Kosher food and all visitors or bags brought into the hospital had to be inspected by security at the main entrance for anything that was considered non-kosher.. As my population of patients picked up and the majority were cancer patients, there was a push to liberalize the Kosher food restriction to cater for the cancer patient and the terminally ill who were also predominantly African American and/or Hispanic.. With petitions and an increasing patient base, kosher food was gradually replaced. Some blamed me for the change but the change was inevitable as Paterson's Jewish population gradually left the city for greener pastures in the suburbs. As the population dynamics changed in Paterson so did the Barnert Hospital. The Jewish doctors also took to the trend and gradually followed their patients. In the late nineteen nineties there was an exodus of the doctors to Valley Hospital in Ridgewood. As the Jewish population dwindled there was left an Asian- Indian population of physicians and suddenly there was an influx of Arab doctors who came from the St. Joseph's teaching programs. They were hired by fellow Arab doctors to attain their green cards in Paterson where working for the poor was considered a criteria for obtaining a green card.. Their numbers swelled in all the departments and gradually took over the majority role in the hospital. Every committee became headed by an Arab. Physicians who did not refer patients to them became targets for suspensions whilst grave complications caused by their colleagues went unchallenged. Emergency room calls became more segregated and the hospital took a downward spiral. It was rumored that St. Joseph's hospital had brought this onslaught in an effort to harm physicians who were resisting take -over attempts by that hospital. The chief of Vascular surgery in St. Joseph's hospital did not only become the chief of surgery but because of the Arab and Indian majority became the President of the Medical Staff. Physicians like me and Dr. P who had the most outpatients and majority of the inpatients came under intense scrutiny. The owners of the Hospital seeing this form of instability and increasing financial losses did not see a need to keep the hospital opened. In September, 2007, the hospital was slated to close without any accommodation made to cater for the numerous patients we still had. The State of New Jersey was unaware of the presents of these patients. After the nursing supervisor and myself had made a call to the state health authorities indicating that the fate of my patients was in danger since no alternative hospital would take the patients that we had, the date of closure was delayed by the state. At this point in order for the hospital to show that it had no patients, Dr. P who was now the President of the medical staff and my competitor and whose office was and still is about a hundred yards from mine and who was also a Medical Executive Committee member of St. Joseph's Hospital decided to suspend the doctors who were still admitting their patients to Barnert Hospital. The reason given for my suspension was that I had not presented a chest X'ray report and my CDS certificate which was due on the thirty first of October was not renewed. On Monday when I presented the said documents to the Medical Staff office, I was told that Dr. P had left for Thailand and did not want the acting

Medical Staff President to take any action. In the meantime he had already paraded all the suspended doctors name to the entire hospital as if we had committed murder. Dr. BB who was the acting President and not Dr. P who was now the Vice President of the Medical Staff and who got into sexual harassment problems and had under gone State Medical Board and Medicare suspensions himself indicated that he could not lift the suspension. After Dr. BB had undergone therapy for sexual harassment issues and returned to Barnert Hospital no doctor on his Arab side wanted him back on staff. I labored and had a plea from the workers and other staff members to give him a chance to redeem himself. He was also the physician for the Passaic County Jail which he had lost during his suspension. It was my patient Mrs. Cook who was one of the Democratic establishment figures who helped him get his job back in the Passaic County jail after it had already given to Dr. E who was also an Arab. The goal of this suspension was to demonstrate to the state that no patients were coming to the hospital to facilitate its closure. Despite requests to follow the hospital's bye-laws which are meant to protect innocent physicians, they were never rendered till the hospital closed in March 2008. When Barnert hospital closed its door St. Joseph's Hospital got an opportunity to punish people like me who for years was resisting its take-over of Barnert hospital. All the medical staff were given privileges as was mandated by the State of New Jersey. They however refused to give me an application for privileges again as they did when I had just ended my fellowship in Hematology and Oncology on the grounds that my Medical Certification in Internal Medicine had just expired. Dr. P who was a member of the Medical Executive committee in conjunction with Dr RA who was involved with a medico-legal issue with a patient of mine over her loss of her voice during a botched ENT surgery decided to block my presence in St. Joseph's. After re-certifying in my Internal Medicine Boards and obtaining a court order by a Passaic County Judge and my case transferred to the labor division of the Passaic Court system through my attorney who suddenly withdrew from my legal case when I could not pay him an additional twenty-five thousand dollars on top of the fifteen thousand dollars he was already paid. It is my understanding that the lawyer has lost his license to practice Law which does not surprise me from the way he handled my case. My wife suspected that he was paid in order to drop my case against St. Joseph's Hospital. I strongly believe that there are institutions who believe they can break laws and get away such as defying a judge's order with impunity. The system is laden with so much falsehood that institutions that now seem to group themselves into medical conglomerates can refuse privileges to competent minorities on the grounds that certain physician are non-conforming rather than not wanting certain ethnic groups into the mix of certain institution. When St. Joseph's hospital refused me privileges and has blocked my ability to get privileges in all the Hospitals in Northern New Jersey, my patients protested by going to their political representatives in Paterson about how the care of cancer patients has been affected by my absence A meeting was held with some of the Councilmen in the Paterson City Council and I was told by Mr, MB who is also the Ombudsman of the hospital that they did not want me because I was not a member of the Italian Mafia. They made up every excuse including that I was not Board Certified which were completely false. Unfortunately in medicine today if you can manage a case differently or do not take orders because you are a black doctor then you are not conforming to the norm as was seen during slavery.. For example the current chief of Medicine one time headed the Medical Ethics Committee of St. Joseph's hospital. The committee around 1997 had declared one of my patients as brain dead without any person on the committee letting me know or informing the patient's family. The family came to me in disgust because all the intravenous fluids and feeding and supportive elements were discontinued without their knowledge or consent. I went to the current Head of Internal Medicine to enquire why I was not given prior information and also why no body from the committee could at least speak to the family. As minority patient s their input in their families well being is not important. If a discussion is held and one has a different view then often is labelled a non-conformist, punished and black-listed by the medical establishment. The healthcare system in this country has to improve for the poor and especially for the blacks and Hispanics who through out slavery was the back bone of medical experimentation and which still goes on today.. In all aspects of medical care management, the black person is behind. Blacks are more likely to get the wrong transfusions, get severe complications and have the highest morbidity and mortality than the average white person. Blacks are more likely to be discharged prematurely than other groups as was recently demonstrated in Mr. Duncan's case when he was sent home when he had the Ebola virus. It did not surprise me that Mr. Duncan died because I had a bet with my family that he was going to die because the care givers were more afraid of the patient than of the disease. Even though blacks make up the majority of the teaching programs they have the highest morbidity and mortality rate than any other groups. The blacks who make up the bulk of our teaching programs have the highest complication rates of procedures performed by residents and fellows either due to lack of supervision or using incompetent teachers solely because they belong to the privileged classes and not because they are qualified or exemplary.. The Obama care program which is coming up is based on expanding the Medicaid program. What it does not take into consideration is that if you give some body a low salary how do you expect them to take care of the same patients one would have preferred not to take care of in the first place.. The Medicaid program that pays a doctor sixteen dollars to see a patient on a Sub-speciality consultation when one has spent countless hours studying and accumulating loans is paid less than somebody snaking a pipe. The hope of Obama care is to redistribute care that does not already exist and a lot of people registering will make a lot of insurance exchanges rich whilst their care continues to labor in prejudice and racism. Is it to help the poor or the rich.?. We await to see that if steps are not taken to remove the canker of racism and inequality in medicine the goal of reducing health care cost and the health budget of this country will remain a dream as we have seen other problems of society that has refused to accept that we are all Gods children.

www.ingramcontent.com/pod-product-compliance
Lightning Source LLC
Chambersburg PA
CBHW030928180526
45163CB00002B/494